PRAISE FOR
REFUGE IN THE STORM

"In a world where crises happen every day, living through disaster and with trauma are frighteningly common human experiences. Caregivers grapple with the crises of their own lives even as they seek to help those actively experiencing crisis and disaster in the present moment.... This book is essential reading; from foundational chapters on dealing with personal loss to wide-scale disasters to very specific situations like the ICU—no matter their circumstance, every caregiver can benefit from each piece."

—MONICA SANFORD, assistant dean of Multireligious Ministry at Harvard University and author of *Kalyanamitra*

"*Refuge in the Storm* is a timely and precious anthology of experienced Buddhist psychologists, chaplains, counselors, and other voices from around the world.... [the essays are] accessible and practical resources for those providing care today to continue their work as bodhisattvas based on the wisdom contained in Buddhist texts. This collection of essays is clearly a gift from bodhisattvas to bodhisattvas."

—VENERABLE JUEWEI, director of the Humanistic Buddhism Center at Nan Tien Institute and ordained in the Fo Guang Shan Buddhist order

"An accessible, practical, scholarly resource for chaplains and other caregivers. *Refuge in the Storm* contextualizes what we know about crisis care by integrating psychosocial understandings and Buddhist wisdom in nuanced and generative ways. This is dāna of the highest order, a foundational text for the maturing profession of Buddhist chaplaincy. You'll want this in your professional library to refer to over and over."

—DUANE BIDWELL, Center for Health Professions Education, Hebert School of Medicine; author of *When One Religion Isn't Enough*; and board member at the Society for Buddhist-Christian Studies

REFUGE
IN
THE
STORM

REFUGE IN THE STORM

BUDDHIST VOICES IN CRISIS CARE

EDITED BY

Nathan Jishin Michon

North Atlantic Books
Huichin, unceded Ohlone land
aka Berkeley, California

"Responding to Multiple Crises and the Roles of Community Chaplaincy" by Dawn Neal is reprinted with permission from the author and the *San Mateo Daily Journal*, September 4, 2020, www.smdailyjournal.com/opinion/guest _perspectives/call-for-a-community-ethic-of-compassion/article_11a5e442-ee47-11ea-8890-6f8bf6d3ad91.html.

"Psycho-Spiritual Relief Work in the Tsunami Areas: An Interview with Rev. Jin Hitoshi," by Jonathan S. Watts, which was adapted from a chapter published in *This Precious Life: Buddhist Tsunami Relief and Anti-Nuclear Activism in Post 3/11 Japan* (Yokohama, Japan: International Buddhist Exchange Center, November 2011), is reprinted with permission.

"The Path to Buddhist Chaplaincy in the U.S." by Jitsujo T. Gauthier, PhD; Daijaku Judith Kinst, PhD; Leigh Miller, PhD; and Elaine Yuen, PhD, was originally published by the Chaplaincy Innovation Lab and is reprinted with permission.

Excerpts from *one long listening: a memoir of grief, friendship, and spiritual care* by Chenxing Han, published by North Atlantic Books, copyright © 2023 by Chenxing Han, are reprinted by permission of North Atlantic Books.

Published by
North Atlantic Books
Huichin, unceded Ohlone land
aka Berkeley, California

Cover art © Anko via Adobe Stock
Cover design by Susan Zucker
Book design by Happenstance Type-O-Rama

Printed in the United States of America

Refuge in the Storm: Buddhist Voices in Crisis Care is sponsored and published by North Atlantic Books, an educational nonprofit based in the unceded Ohlone land Huichin (*aka* Berkeley, CA) that collaborates with partners to develop cross-cultural perspectives; nurture holistic views of art, science, the humanities, and healing; and seed personal and global transformation by publishing work on the relationship of body, spirit, and nature.

North Atlantic Books' publications are distributed to the US trade and internationally by Penguin Random House Publisher Services. For further information, visit our website at www.northatlanticbooks.com.

Library of Congress Cataloging-in-Publication Data
Names: Michon, Nathan Jishon, compiler.
Title: Refuge in the storm : Buddhist voices in crisis care / Nathan Jishin
 Michon.
Description: Berkeley, California : North Atlantic Books, [2022] | Includes
 index. | Summary: "A tool for care providers to navigate through
 suffering and healing, Nathan Jishin Michon compiles a wide range of
 Buddhist perspectives on crisis care. Michon brings 24 essays written by
 different people from various backgrounds and professions that support
 and guide readers through individual and collective crises by harnessing
 the power of compassion, mindfulness, and Buddhist wisdom"— Provided by
 publisher.
Identifiers: LCCN 2022045188 | ISBN 9781623178093 (trade paperback) | ISBN
 9781623178109 (ebook)
Subjects: LCSH: Caring—Religious aspects—Buddhism. | Social
 service—Religious aspects—Buddhism. | Crisis management—Religious
 aspects—Buddhism. | Spiritual life—Buddhism.
Classification: LCC BQ4570.C27 R44 2022 | DDC 294.3/444—dc23/eng/20221215
LC record available at https://lccn.loc.gov/20

1 2 3 4 5 6 7 8 9 KPC 27 26 25 24 23

This book includes recycled material and material from well-managed forests. North Atlantic Books is committed to the protection of our environment. We print on recycled paper whenever possible and partner with printers who strive to use environmentally responsible practices.

CONTENTS

ACKNOWLEDGMENTS

I first want to thank all the authors who participated in this project, lending their expertise and wisdom. In particular, I want to thank Chenxing Han, who helped with some organizational aspects of the volume. I also want to thank those who helped spread the original call for papers around the world. The response when this book was in the initial planning stages was incredible, but could not have happened without those who helped transmit its message. I was unsure if this book would really take off the way it did, but the number of responses to that original call for papers was almost overwhelming. In particular, I would also like to thank Sumi Loundon Kim, who offered some initial feedback on the project and recommended authors. I also want to thank my parents, who helped proofread initial drafts of some chapters. Moreover, I want to extend gratitude toward my teachers, both in care and Buddhist studies, as well as Dharma teachers—I am indebted to the countless lessons you all provided and dedicate any merit from the efforts of this book to the well-being of sentient beings.

FIVE IRISES FOR MARY OLIVER
(1935–2019)

By Mushim Ikeda

—for k.o.
1.25.2019

I brought home five irises from the grocery store
and when they unfurled
felt the pleasure of their color

moist flags stained like winter sky
right after the sun sets, fierce cobalt, then
cold and with it, sadness.

This is not startling and original.
The poet Mary Oliver said this is okay
enough and it is okay enough

to be simple and happy for awhile.
We aren't always reduced
to our entangled thoughts, our anguish.

Praying with my friend this morning, he said
Thank you, he asked *Help* —
we bow down and rise up.

O help us now, Beloved Friend, to meet
our worst fears, the suffering on this planet
with the brief bright faces

of cut flowers opening, with the perfume oils
of coffee, the sturdy clay of the cup,
the clock tick it takes to say the one word love.

INTRODUCTION
Buddhist Crisis Care

Nathan Jishin Michon, MDiv, PhD

T he local train chugged along its route, cityscapes gradually fading into the surrounding nature and small towns. Exiting at a small station, I went to deposit my ticket in a typical electronic stall, but found none. Only a small box that trusted passengers to insert a ticket with the proper fee stood barely noticeable before the workerless exit. Rural Japan was always so safe and trusting. That thought came over me while walking through the train station into this small city for the first time. Yet, the feeling was conflicting, with some opposing internal sensations. For one, I now needed to navigate myself to a place I'd never been without anyone available to ask for directions. I'm grateful for cell phones and their satellite maps, but still prefer some human interaction when entering new and unfamiliar whereabouts.

Another reason for some consternation, however, was quite different. This was no normal trip and no normal area to visit. This was the town of Ishinomaki. Several years earlier, this town was near the epicenter of one of history's largest-ever recorded earthquakes, sparking a devastatingly immense tsunami. Although years had passed and no signs of destruction remained visible from the station, it was hard not to feel some of the gravity of the events that had transpired on this land I was just stepping foot on. Many families and individuals were still in temporary housing units as the area continued its recovery. I was heading toward a community center in the midst of those units. It was my first day as a volunteer chaplain with a group that regularly arranged events to care for the people there.

When I arrived at the housing units, I had to wander a while searching for the community center. I was relieved when I finally saw the sign of the volunteer organization: Café de Monk. It was a play on words using the English *monk* and the Japanese *monku,* meaning "to complain." Thus, it was a place where people could come and complain about aspects of their life to the monks (or other volunteers) if they felt so inclined. However, it aimed to be a relaxed and pressure-free oasis. Volunteers provided attendees with complimentary drinks and snacks, along with group tables and activities to help facilitate a sense of community among them. Then, only if they wished to talk about their pain, volunteer chaplains and listeners were on hand to hear their stories and accompany them through the retelling of their tragedies.

As I entered, volunteers were already bustling about, finishing some of the setup, and attendees had seemingly begun to arrive and take their seats. I saw the head of the organization walking briskly about and directing others. He looked busy, so I figured I'd stand to the side and wait until he had a moment. Or maybe someone else would make themselves apparent as another leader and I could ask them how I could help in the setup. The scene was both exciting and slightly overwhelming as people hurried about the room with what appeared to be some last-minute arrangements. People looked generally cheerful and happy to meet each other there. I heard plenty of thick local dialect and quietly hoped my Japanese would be adequate to communicate in this setting.

A woman approached me. Recognizing me as a foreigner in my *samue* clothing, the informal working clothes regularly worn by Buddhist priests, she asked if I came as a volunteer chaplain. I was a little relieved someone approached me rather than having to interrupt anyone. I looked forward to beginning to help out with setup or in some other capacity. "Yes," I replied. "I look forward to the experience today. Is there anything I can do to help?" "Well . . ." she answered with a short pause, "I used to live in one of the small villages on the coast. The tsunami took half the people there and most of the people I knew. My parents survived, but being stuck with only them and the other elderly people here, it is so lonely. After all this time, I still just feel overwhelmed by the grief . . ." Of course, soon after her story began, I quickly realized this was not a fellow volunteer. But the suddenness of her story and my unfamiliarity in the new surroundings caught me quite off guard. I had been relaxing into the energy of the room while dealing with a slight sensory overload in the very new environment.

I was not at all present in my body or with my feelings. I was definitely not at all prepared for that sort of story in that moment.

I quickly tried to snap myself into a care type of mindset. *Get into chaplain mode now,* I told myself. *Where are my body and mind right now? Be aware of them. Breathe. Slow that breathing pace down. Let myself be calmer. Bring my attention more fully to the person speaking in front of me. Let that sense of compassion arise.* I tried to tell myself all these things in the split seconds around her words. But the reality of the mental and physical transition was not nearly as instantaneous as those internal instructions I was thinking.

Honestly, I am very sure I wasn't the very best version of myself as a care provider in the moments that followed, but I continued to listen to her story as compassionately as I could and tried to *be* with her through the greatest presence I could muster. The experience, however, also served as an impeccable reminder about mindful vigilance, especially when entering a space of disaster or other crisis situations.

Being in or entering into a crisis situation can be nerve-racking, unsettling, and exhausting as well as rewarding, invigorating, and uplifting. There can be a broad mix of internal reactions as we wade through an environment of unpredictable churning and dynamic energies. However, it is important to be prepared to face those situations before entering. You want to be a skilled swimmer before jumping into the deep end of the wave pool. This volume is not meant to be the end-all be-all of such preparation, but at least a starting point or a supplement to practical training available elsewhere. As part of a tradition built on the questions of transcending or overcoming suffering, Buddhists in crisis care have plenty of wisdom to offer with some unique perspectives and insights adapted from their traditional wisdom to address issues faced by those struggling through life's crises. Café de Monk, the organization described above, is only one example of a Buddhist group deeply engaged in such work.

The oasis-like refuge provided by Café de Monk also serves as a wonderful symbol for this volume. *Refuge* is a vitally important idea in Buddhism. In ancient India, it was associated with allegiance to a king or kingdom because of the security they provided. In Buddhism, we use the notion of refuge because commitment to awakening, the Dharma teachings, and the teachers and community who support that teaching are said to provide the deepest form of security for our hearts and minds—a sacred refuge. As Victor Gabriel explains in chapter 1, the vows associated with these refuges help us connect with ourselves, our community, and our reality. By first establishing that refuge within ourselves, we can more readily be available to provide refuge to others.

This collection of chapters began assembling in the midst of the 2020 pandemic as borders shut down around the world, but the conversation invited a broad range of discussion around different forms of crises occurring. The original call for papers for this volume left the word *crisis* undefined purposely to welcome openness and conversation around the multitude of crises occurring in the world for various populations. This book describes options for helping others—and ourselves—in dealing with a wide range of crises that occur within our lives and the world around us, including the struggles with the pandemic, debilitating forms of illness, the dying process, personal relationships, racial injustice, immigration, fracturing society, and natural disasters. Authors are experienced chaplains, nurses, medical technicians, psychologists, professors, and others who offer a treasure trove of experience and wisdom to this volume.

First, though, this introduction will set the stage by defining some key terms in crisis care, introducing a few key pieces of literature, and showing how Buddhist notions fit within some broader principles of crisis care. It will then provide some tips for spiritual first aid during disasters. Next, it briefly introduces the psychological and physical processes that occur during trauma and severe stress that often occur during crisis. It will then show how Buddhist notions and practices around compassion and kindness can play a role in mitigating such effects. Finally, this chapter will provide a detailed introduction to the chapters that lie ahead in the volume.

Crises and Disasters

Crises can be natural or human-caused and may differ widely in scale and duration. A disaster is typically a larger-scale term for crisis, but sometimes the words are interchangeable. In a broad sense, we can define *crisis* as a disruptive event or relationship. The American Red Cross defines a disaster as "an event of such destructive magnitude and force as to dislocate, injure, or kill people, separate family members, and damage or destroy homes." Rabbi Stephen Roberts and Rev. Willard W. C. Ashley Sr. also add that disasters can overwhelm the initial coping capacities and resources for an individual, a family, or a community. Disaster disruptions can be spiritual, emotional, economic, physical, and ecological. . . . Disasters produce a ripple effect. The number of individuals affected by a disaster and in need of spiritual care is often dramatically greater than the number of people killed or injured.[1]

In terror attacks, for example, studies show up to ten times the number of mental health victims for every physically injured person.[2] No matter the scale of a crisis, we should be aware of the way its effects can ripple out to ourselves and others with any connection to it.

Care can occur in many forms, as the following chapters will show, but for those of us who are Buddhists or identify with another spiritual path, we may be particularly well-positioned to provide spiritual care. In this sense, *spiritual* typically refers to a person's path to find meaning in life or comprehending their life experiences. The mission of disaster spiritual care, according to Roberts and Ashley,

> is to provide appropriate short-term and long-term care for people who have been affected by both the initial trauma and the ongoing disaster situation. The goal is to provide sensitive spiritual and emotional care to affected individuals and families by respecting a person's culture, religious tradition, and faith commitments. . . . The role of the spiritual care provider in a disaster is not to shelter people or to help them escape, but to help those affected draw upon their own emotional and spiritual resources in the midst of their pain. Our goal is not necessarily to take away their grief, but to help them work through their grief.[3]

In the United States, one key organization uniting efforts in disaster care, particularly noted for its inclusion of faith-based organizations, is National Voluntary Organizations Active in Disaster (NVOAD). They value "communication, coordination, collaboration, and cooperation" while hoping to organize the diverse efforts of numerous volunteer groups to ensure that different people's efforts are well-rounded in providing for many people's needs, especially in the context of larger disaster sites.

Because of NVOAD's large contingent of faith-based volunteer organizations, they have also been a leader in disaster spiritual care resources. They developed a document called "Points of Consensus" on disaster spiritual care that provides guiding ethics to those from any religious organization volunteering with NVOAD and have been influential in other disaster volunteer organizations. They also produced several longer documents to help guide the spiritual care of religious volunteers during crisis situations. One of the organization's members produced the volume *Light Our Way*, which is "the first major publication accepted and endorsed by the wide-ranging and diverse scope of faith groups active at the time within NVOAD." Roberts's and Ashley's edited volume *Disaster Spiritual Care* is an excellent guide to many points on the theme. Written from Jewish and Christian perspectives, the volume includes a multipoint "Key Principles of Disaster Spiritual Care,"[4] which in many ways is a summary of the primary themes of the book. While describing the twelve principles here, I weave more of a Buddhist perspective through the commentary.

Buddhist Disaster and Crisis Care

1. *Basic needs come first. Particularly in the immediate hours and days after a disaster, before helping with the spiritual needs of those affected, assess that the person you are working with is not hungry, has access to and has taken any medications that they normally require, and has a safe place to sleep. Most people are unable to focus on spiritual issues when their basic physical needs are in doubt.*

This is especially true in natural disasters but may apply to many other crises when people lack basic needs. Basic needs are the priority. In any situation, we must ensure that people's basic needs are met well before inquiring about their various spiritual needs. There may be many layers of suffering, but things like food, water, and safety are at a fundamental level that must be addressed before we can explore other forms of suffering. Sometimes, even if food and drink are available, people can forget to eat or dehydrate themselves without thinking during a crisis—a simple question and offer can bring this to light. During disasters that require hasty evacuation of homes, people might forget about or have a depleted supply of necessary medications as well, which further complicates already complex situations. The body and mind are integrally connected in all we do during our human lives. Well before people can even come to terms with mental and emotional issues or even begin processing them, we must first simply ensure they are supplied with basic needs that allow for later processing to occur.

2. *Do no harm.*

The ideals of ahimsa are commonly recognized in Buddhism. Yet we must try to consistently use Right Effort and Right Mindfulness to apply those regularly, and this is not easy in the midst of any crisis. We have to observe ourselves and try to find those ways that work to remind us to stay on the path and not forget our own well-being in the process. A lack of selfhood is a foundational truth in Buddhism. Under the interconnection this concept refers to, it is very clear that ignorance to our own well-being during a disaster could ultimately be harmful to others in many ways. We must remember to be kind to both our own bodies and minds as well as others. Many Chinese temples regularly post the phrase that covers three points of the Eightfold Path, a fundamental Buddhist teaching: think good thoughts, speak good words, and do good deeds. Our thoughts, speech, and action all have potential to be either harmful or helpful in myriad ways. Especially during crises, it is important to observe those effects and pay attention to ways we can either help or, at least, not further complicate a situation.

3. *Each person you work with is unique and holy.*

Buddhists might not think of "holy" as the first word to use, but I believe we can understand the intent. All people are unique and special in their own way. We have to respect those differences and be attuned to each person's individual proclivities and needs. While it is still very important to learn from previous experience, we cannot allow that knowledge to obscure each new moment, new face, and new needs that we encounter. From a Mahāyāna Buddhist perspective, we might say that we should honor the Buddha in every individual. Those from the Zen school use the phrase "beginner's mind" as a way to emphasize the mind-state required to recognize the unique qualities of each new person in each new moment.

4. *Do not proselytize, evangelize, exploit, or take advantage of those affected by a disaster, and don't allow others to do so.*

Those in the midst of any crisis or disaster situation are extremely vulnerable. They often do not even have the mental capacity for proper consent to engage in religious discussions. The Dharma may be critical as our own pedestal and it might inform our actions, but we must maintain focus on each individual's own needs in front of us. As good as our intentions may be and as much as we may love the Dharma, it is important not to assume (even unintentionally) what is best for the person in front of us. Even if not trying to explicitly convert another to our belief structure, we might still unintentionally speak overtly from our own faith perspective. As much as possible, it is good to use the terms and viewpoint of people's own identified faith traditions—or find someone else who can—especially if the person so requests. In Buddhism, the primary concern is ending or reducing suffering. There is no requirement that it has to be done in a specifically "Buddhist" way. So, I think the tradition naturally lends itself to prioritizing other people's needs and meeting them where they are. Sadly, however, it is not uncommon for people from various religious traditions, including Buddhists, to proselytize during disasters. It is important to be aware of potential instances around us and possibly find skillful ways to intercede in order to ensure that people have the space they need, without external pressures, to grieve and process in their own way and in a way in which they themselves are comfortable.

5. *Respect the spiritual, religious, and cultural diversity of those you are working with—ask questions about things you do not understand. Grief, both short- and long-term, looks different in different cultures and religions—ask before you assume.*

It is almost always better to ask about something we don't know rather than guess or make an assumption regarding things with which we are unfamiliar. People are generally open about answering basic questions about their religion and culture, especially when we are genuinely trying to help them. In disasters these issues are particularly pertinent if people have lost loved ones. Handling death and tragedy can differ greatly depending on one's religion and culture. Even the same religion or the same sect can be practiced quite differently within different cultures. So it is imperative to keep an open mind. Helping them grieve or find the resources they need to do so may involve learning and asking numerous questions. In her book *Cultural Competence in Trauma Therapy: Beyond the Flashback,* Laura S. Brown states:

> Responding to trauma in a culturally competent manner requires the [caregiver] to understand how those added meanings that derive from context and identity make each instance of trauma unique. It also requires the [caregiver's] awareness of her or his own identities, biases, and participations in

cultural hierarchies of power and privilege, powerlessness and disadvantage, as well as personal experiences of trauma. Failure to bring cultural competence to the table can lead to missteps in genuinely helping trauma survivors, or worse can result in deepening the wounds of trauma, creating secondary and tertiary traumas that are more painful than the original because they are correctly appraised by victims and survivors as unnecessary wounds.[5]

Balancing compassion with wisdom is always important for skillful action. Of course, we cannot learn everything about everyone's potential background, but engaging in what trainings we can in advance is often helpful. Being aware of the areas of our own ignorance and kindly asking to learn more about another are always safer than making assumptions about others.

6. *Presence—meet the person you are working with wherever they may be in their spiritual and religious life. Accept them as they are and where they are.*

In Buddhist traditions, we have many tools at our hands to enhance our capacity to be present and provide presence to others. Mindfulness is part of the Noble Eightfold Path, but in naming those parts of the path, the Buddha also distinguished between "right mindfulness" and "wrong mindfulness." Numerous times in the sutras, he describes *right* mindfulness as combining mindfulness with ardency and alertness. Mindfulness, or *sati,* refers to remembering the task at hand. *Sampajañña,* the word for "alertness," refers more to the aspect of awareness related to what is happening in body and mind while that focus is taking place. The third part of this equation, as Thānissaro Bhikkhu states, refers to "being intent on what you're doing, trying your best to do it skillfully. This doesn't mean that you have to keep straining and sweating all the time, just that you're continuous in developing skillful habits and abandoning unskillful ones."[6]

This is important to keep in mind while we are with anyone going through a crisis. Our attention while with them is not blind. We likely recognize the need for combining our mindfulness with loving-kindness, compassion, and equanimity in those moments. We pay attention to their subtle verbal and nonverbal cues, how they react to our own words, gestures, and expressions. With those observations, we adjust while learning moment to moment, inferring about the unspoken subtle needs of the person or people before us. To accept that individual for who they are is also accepting the different ways they can be changing themselves from moment to moment. During a crisis, these shifts can happen far more often and more drastically than at other times. To be with another through that dance and ride the storm with them can also sometimes help bring that boat more safely to shore.

7. Help victims and survivors tell their story.

Keep in mind that in the very immediate aftermath of any crisis or disaster, victims might not be ready to share their story, and it should not be forced in any way until that person is ready on their own terms. However, when they are ready and want to express that story, we can be there with them. Practice active and reflective listening. You can do this by asking clarifying questions at parts of the story, or repeating, paraphrasing, or trying to sum up pieces of their story every so often. For example, "So you were so concerned for your parents' welfare, you are only now realizing the toll this experience took on your own well-being." This offers them the opportunity not only to know they are being heard, but also potentially sparks more details they'd like to add. Or they may make corrections or adjustments or other clarifying points to their own story. Especially for people going through crises, stories are rarely linear. They may go back and forth in time or jump to relationships with other people and places. What is important is that we accompany them through this process.

I personally like to internally practice *mettā* (loving-kindness) meditation while listening to people's stories. This is a way to quietly dig into the resources of my own tradition without imposing them on the other, a way that helps me listen more deeply without interruption. I combine this with imagery of light, imagining the light of my loving-kindness reaching, stretching out from me, and encompassing both of us during that time. It can take practice, but this helps me both monitor my own body and mind while also paying close attention to the other and maintaining a compassionate and open mindset. I adjust the visualization depending on my own feelings and energy level at the time of the interaction. For example, there may be times when I don't feel as good for whatever reason; then, I imagine that energy reaching them from the cosmos or some point in space rather than my own body. If I am tired, rather than imagining the light encompassing their whole body, I may have a reduced focus: maybe on only their head or heart area, or some area they mentioned needs healing.

You may adjust with practices or prayers from your own tradition and see what works for you. It is simply important that the practice *complement* rather than *impede* your presence as a listener.

8. *Be aware of confidentiality.*

This is typically made clear for employees, but not as often for volunteers. Be sure you are fully aware of any rules or procedures around confidentiality regarding the capacity in which you are serving. During some disasters, numerous fields are mixed together in a setting and each contributing organization may have slightly different rules. It is good to confirm workers' and volunteers' understanding around confidentiality before meeting the victims or patients. Know that when others share their story with you, it remains their story. It deserves the utmost respect. There are times when you must share aspects of what they say with a medical professional or psychologist to assist in their healing process. But otherwise, keep the details to yourself. If you share aspects of someone's story with other care providers for learning purposes, be sure not to disclose any identifying details of the individual whose case you are describing.

9. *Make neither promises nor something that even sounds like a promise.*

In the Abhaya Sutra, the Buddha offered a checklist of three questions to ensure a statement was actually "right speech." (a) Is it truthful? (b) Is it beneficial? (c) Is it timely? Sometimes speech may be true and beneficial, but not at the right time. Sometimes speech can be timely and beneficial, but not true. Speech must fulfill all three qualifications to be "right speech." When helping someone in trouble, many people are tempted to say, "I promise you'll be OK." But how do you know that? These statements are often made with the best intent but have potential to backfire in either the short term or long term. A person in a deep state of suffering and stress may not see an end in sight. They could be angry at your confident assumption that they'll get through it. They may think, *You don't really know me or what I've been through. How can you say that?* Even if a promise offers short-term consolation, it can backfire if the promise is not soon met. "You said I'd be OK, and I'm still not close to OK!" Particularly in disaster situations, when circumstances and resource availability can change rapidly, promises may be particularly difficult to keep. Instead, consider statements in the present tense or referencing an action you will take, like "I am here with you." "I will try to find you a bandage right away."

10. *Be sensitive to language barriers. Remember that it is often difficult to express yourself effectively in a second language. If possible, provide spiritual care in the person's native language by finding a spiritual care provider who speaks their language. Allow the person or family you are working with to choose their own translator. Ideally, do not use children as an interpreter, though it is sometimes necessary to do so.*

People speaking in their nonnative language have a wide range in their level of comfort with second or third languages. Moreover, it is almost always more challenging to listen or speak in other languages during high-stress situations. Even if you find trouble communicating with someone, recognize how much you can convey through your facial expressions and gestures. As Shushin R. A. Peterson expresses in chapter 15, there are many examples of Zen koans that show how much meaning can truly be expressed in a few words or less. Maintaining a calm inner sense and sharing a moment with compassion toward someone may still make a large difference in assuaging their anxieties before you go to find a translator or care provider who can communicate with them.

11. *Remember when working with immigrants that both legal and illegal immigrants often fear or distrust the government due to their life circumstances.*

This is an important reminder, especially if you are working or volunteering in connection to a government service. Even if you do not directly work for the government, you may still be indirectly associated with them through your position. There can be strong fears, doubts, distrust, or other reactions when bringing someone to a government-run facility, such as a temporary shelter. Fear or distrust directed toward you may not be personal at all. In Buddhism, we often hear the phrase "causes and conditions" as a reminder of how detailed and intertwined the various strings of conditionality really are. An individual may have migrated from a land where they or their relatives were tortured and abused by government officials. A person may have been brought to the country without proper paperwork and always told to avoid government workers as they were raised. We never truly know all the background another has gone through. It is important to keep an open mind and open heart in dealing with all people, but to be especially aware of these issues when caring for immigrants and some of the unique concerns they may have.

12. *Practice active listening—listen with your ears, eyes, and heart. Do far less talking than you do listening. Never respond with, "I know how you feel," or, "You think that is bad; let me tell you my story."*

As the latter statement indicates, we must be careful with our words while listening to others' feelings and stories. How can we truly know what another feels? Saying that we *know* how another feels can be very off-putting to those going through what feels like a dreadful and unique experience. Likewise, we should not compare experiences. The focus should be on the care seeker and their story. When listening, we listen as much as possible with our entire being. The following excerpt from Thich Nhat Hanh's *Chanting from the Heart*'s verse on "Loving Speech and Deep Listening" beautifully reflects several aspects of an embodied view of Buddhist listening, and its recitation can be a wonderful developmental practice in itself:

> I shall practice diligently
> to guard my body and mind
> with conscious breathing
> and through awareness of my steps,
> so that I can embrace
> the anger and irritation in my heart;
> so I can sit and listen deeply
> with all my compassion
> and so the other person has a chance to share
> all their hidden suffering.
> I want to learn to listen deeply
> with sincere loving-kindness
> so that the other person can suffer less. . . .

The passage indicates the aspects of self-care valuable in preparation for deep listening. This embodied approach is especially suitable for listening to another with one's whole self.

While all these points are good to keep in mind, what can we do in the very immediate aftermath of a crisis? Those with specific medical or psychological training have particular roles to play. But for most others, there are a few steps to spiritual first aid which can help provide people with some foundational presence and care before they may receive more specialized attention elsewhere.

Spiritual First Aid

Reverend Julie Taylor, chaplain and former executive director of New York's Disaster Chaplaincy Services, explains that spiritual first aid is a "crisis intervention technique used during times of acute stress. As the name implies, it is first aid, not a cure, not fixing."[7] She bases her model off the International Critical Incident Stress Foundation's (ICISF) Pastoral Crisis Intervention Program, and it is intended for the immediate aftermath of a crisis or "critical incident." Especially in the case of disaster situations, it is also important to emphasize we should avoid acting alone. As much as we may want to jump in and help, many individuals acting on their own during a disaster situation can lead to disorganized and uneven care—efforts may end up ignoring those who need it most or even cause unintended harm. Many larger organizations will likely be on the scene, and getting connected first through them, you can play a vital role as part of a broader team of helpers.

Taylor introduces five basic stages for spiritual first aid: (1) stabilization and introduction, (2) acknowledgment, (3) facilitating understanding, (4) encouraging adaptive coping, and (5) referral as needed. The first step is to be a calming presence while introducing your name and role, along with an offer of assistance. For example, "Hello. My name is Nathan, a chaplain and disaster aid volunteer. Do you need a blanket?" You might be offering water, a snack, or other basic needs depending on the circumstances. These opening moments of communication also offer opportunities for immediate assessment. You may need to call for a translator, doctor, or psychologist immediately in certain cases. The goal is to be a stable pillar of presence during a person's time of need if they want companionship or a firm psychoemotional foundation to grasp onto during those critical initial moments.

The second stage is acknowledging their situation. Listen attentively to what they say and ask questions to help you understand their situation and needs. They may not be ready to tell their story, and you should not pressure them to do so. During the immediate aftermath, many people are not yet ready to process what happened and simply need to feel safe and secure again. However, if they want to speak, you can be there to listen to that story. As Taylor states, "the goal of spiritual first aid is not to get to the bottom of the trauma or crisis . . . but to mitigate the effects of the crisis and refer the individual on to a higher level if needed."[8] You can acknowledge, however, any shock or terror they express. They may express their state of mind directly or indirectly through their words, have a quivering voice, or be visibly shaking.

Next, it is important to facilitate basic understanding of the person's experience. You can reassure them that any unusual feelings or reactions—notions that they are not acting like themselves—are common occurrences. *Common* is generally a better word to use than *normal* in these situations. *Normal* and *abnormal* are psychological terms that can have therapeutic implications and misunderstandings. To call one person "normal" while the person next to them has different feelings and reactions can induce discomfort in such situations. *Common* is seen as a generally safer term. The main task, though, is to help facilitate their understanding of their own reactions to the situation. This can involve numerous questions. Try to be *inquisitive* without being *invasive* while maintaining a gentle voice and presence.

The fourth step is encouraging adaptive coping. Based on what you have heard in their responses, you may recommend a couple of strategies to help them navigate the crisis at hand. The strategies offered, of course, should be based on their response and communication in the previous steps. Try to offer something that is fitting for their own needs in that moment. If the individual has a strong faith in a particular tradition and is receptive to prayer, you may offer to pray with them. Or perhaps offer one or two examples of a breathing practice. You may even take some breaths with them.

Finally, you may want to refer the individual to someone else who can more directly meet their particular needs. In providing spiritual first aid, your main roles are to provide immediate attention, conduct a fundamental assessment, and then connect individuals to other specialists they may need. Thus, it is important to be connected beforehand to various local community members who can meet certain potential needs. If you are volunteering with a larger organization such as the International Committee of the Red Cross, there are many internal possibilities of referral. While listening, you may learn they need immediate mental-health or physician attention. Be prepared to act and contact the necessary individual as the need arises. Sometimes, an individual may require temporary housing or financial assistance. Other times, a person may need someone from their religious tradition to help in the grieving or memorial process. As a stabilizing point for someone in crisis, listening to their immediate concerns, you can help connect them to the specialists they most need in that moment.

Going through any crisis or disaster can have myriad immense challenges. The suffering can be seriously exacerbated by loneliness. Yet, offering to be with those suffering through such experiences in a supportive way can make all the difference. Those who feel supported by others after trauma not only have an easier path to recovery, they often turn around and help others as well. Psychologists refer to this as altruism born of suffering. As Jamil Zaki states,

> When survivors help others, they also help themselves. "Victims" are often stereotyped as weakened by trauma, but many emerge stronger and more fulfilled. "Post-traumatic growth" [PTG]—including greater spirituality, stronger relationships, and a renewed sense of purpose—is almost as common as PTSD.[9]

After surviving the holocaust, Viktor Frankl wrote that someone "who becomes conscious of the responsibility he bears toward a human being . . . will never be able to throw his life away. He knows the 'why' for his existence, and will be able to bear almost any 'how.'"[10]

Of course, trauma and pain are almost never invited guests at the mind's table. Once a crisis has occurred, though, to grow is certainly the more ideal path. The pointers above and all the specific wisdom offered in the chapters that follow can all be tools to help in that journey. But to understand how the mind can teeter between states like PTSD and PTG, it is also helpful to understand some basic functions of the mind and its stress reactions. Understanding those functions can help us better understand both our own reactions and the reactions of others.

Fight, Flight . . . or Flourish

Crises are drastic situations that can often trigger the "fight or flight" stimulus throughout the cells in our bodies. Especially a person who has just witnessed loved ones perishing in a natural disaster or has gone into a complete psychological "flight" mode while escaping a traumatic scene is not acting within their normal state of consciousness. Even otherwise kind and caring people can commit cold or senseless acts when they feel completely overwhelmed. This is important to remember in terms of crisis care. The selfish reactions that some have are not their total selves; the person you see in that moment may not be their regular self. They may need help—and time—to return to who they are.

Essentially, nearly all our survival mechanisms can be categorized into two responses: growth and protection. The fight-or-flight mechanisms fall under the area of "protection." As human beings developed, it was natural to devote all of our bodies' energy to protection responses when danger was imminent. Of course, fleeing or staving off a hungry tiger would be of more immediate importance than philosophizing or even fighting internal disease. Significant stress and fear sets off a chain reaction inside the body that leads to the release of adrenal hormones. This gives people the immediate strength they might need in their musculature, but it has numerous noteworthy side effects: the extra blood that flows to the arms and legs comes at the expense of much of the blood flow to the internal organs. Digestion and absorption processes are interrupted, halting the body's production of energy reserves, the immune system nearly shuts down, and blood flow and hormones in the head are directed to the back of the brain rather than to the front.

Why is this particularly important to consider during crises and disasters? The blood has been diverted from the slower, methodical logic and reasoning sections of the forebrain to the instinctive hindbrain, which controls quick reflexes. The stress and fear can literally create a temporary reduction in people's intelligence, reasoning, and conscious awareness.[11] There are times when rear-brain functions are important during disasters, but other times they can be severely disruptive. Blood flow in the forebrain and the objective reasoning necessary to work through challenges go hand in hand. Being aware of those differences within our own bodies can be incredibly beneficial while trying to operate or help others.

The paths from our brains to the rest of the cells in our bodies are traversed by many little chemical elements called neuropeptides, nicknamed the "molecules of emotion" by Candace Pert, the Georgetown Medical School professor who helped discover them. According to Pert, our bodies are addicted to emotions. Emotions are not just psychological; they are made up of innumerable biochemical reactions. Our hypothalamus produces a blitz of neuropeptides every time we experience emotion. These peptides are assembled according to each emotion and sent racing throughout the body. They latch onto cells that each contain thousands of receptors for peptides. When the peptides lock into each cell, they send signals into it that ultimately create the physical sensations we feel with each emotion.

A critical juncture comes when those cells divide, because the new cells then have more receptors designed to receive peptides from those emotions. Nutrients and drugs such as heroin use these same receptors. The extent of the addiction may differ, but the fact is that the cells of our bodies lead us to crave those chemicals that contain more receptors of a certain type. Although we might consider depression and anger to be negative experiences, they also provide an emotional rush that compounds and leads to more of those emotions. *Awareness of our emotions,* however, can help ebb the tide, and conscious effort toward desirable emotions can help us develop productive patterns.

Other research even shows the power that conscious thought has over our entire genetic structure. Genes are not activated without environmental stimuli. The genes of our chromosomes are covered by proteins. When the proteins receive external signals, they change shape and allow the genetic sequence they were covering to be activated. No matter what genes one might have received from their parents, conscious attention to thoughts and feelings can help control which of those genes are actually activated. Scientists have developed the concept of neuroplasticity, essentially the ability of the brain to change its own hardwiring. Different areas of the brain can grow, and connections that were once solid can change. The overarching theme of these concepts is that conscious thought and attention can change even our longtime mental patterns. If we learn to become more aware of those emotions and how we respond in different situations, we can gain more control over them. Our bodies can then have the space they need to process and heal.

When dealing with those in any crisis, care providers can benefit from an ability to write and rewrite their own reaction and response styles, the way they feel in particular circumstances, and the manner in which they deal with emotions they encounter. Pert compares this effort to changing direction while controlling a sailboat. When we shift the sail to another side, we might not change directions instantly. We may have to wait for the wind to pick up and catch the sail. It will take more energy and effort at first, but if we keep the sail held firm in the new direction long enough, we will soon be sailing smoothly on our new course.

Crisis situations can be intensely challenging but can also offer an opportunity in some ways. The severe intensity on our systems can provide changes that are far quicker than normal. Proper awareness or support can harness the energy of a crisis to promote positive psychological shifts, such as post-traumatic growth.

Besides considering how such data relates to those we care for, we also must be sure to think about how it relates to our own well-being when caring for numerous victims of trauma and crisis. One important further consideration is the type of compassion or empathy we might generate toward others we are working with.

Compassion Fatigue

The term *compassion fatigue* came into use during the 1990s, especially through the writing of Charles Figley. It is closely related to other terms, like *secondary trauma,* and refers to a common condition across caring professions in which continued work with victims of traumatic events leads to physical, emotional, or spiritual fatigue and exhaustion. It is often caused by not properly defining one's own limits or setting appropriate boundaries with relation to the care they provide. As Jamil Zaki states,

> Secondary trauma often gives way to burnout, a much greater proportion than in other branches of medicine. Empathetic professionals bear the brunt of these problems. They become depressed more often than their less empathetic peers, and they are more likely to blame themselves when patients worsen or die.[12]

A list of possible symptoms of compassion fatigue is lengthy and can include: chronic tardiness that had not previously been an issue, depression, decreased joy or happiness, decreased enjoyment of career, decreased concentration, diminished sense of purpose, extreme fatigue, frequent headaches, hypertension, hypervigilance, increased substance abuse, lack of interest in intimacy, lower self-esteem, mood swings, outbursts of anger or rage, regular blaming of self and others, regularly experiencing images of others' traumas even outside the situation, shift in eating habits, thoughts of self-harm, trouble sleeping or frequent nightmares, and workaholism.

As Stephen Roberts, Kevin Ellers, and John Wilson emphasize, compassion fatigue is very responsive to treatment, and anyone who believes they are experiencing it should seek immediate professional help with a person experienced in the field. They particularly recommend the Accelerated Recovery Program (ARP), developed in 1997. But there may be numerous other resources available that are worth looking into, depending on your profession or organization.[13]

The reality of compassion fatigue can often put those from the caring professions in a difficult position. Do you open your heart to your work and leave yourself vulnerable to the psychological effects of all the devastation you face on a daily basis, or close yourself down and disconnect from the emotional experiences of others, becoming less empathetic? Buddhism, of course, offers a middle way. *The type of compassion matters.* And, as will be discussed later, pairing it with equanimity-based practices helps add a defense that allows us to compassionately face suffering while minimizing the associated adverse effects.

Healthy Compassion and Karuna

Western books often point out that *compati,* the Latin root of the word *compassion,* means to "suffer together." Buddhists deeply value compassion, but the ultimate goal of Buddhism is to *transcend suffering.* So how are these views reconciled? We should remember that compassion in the Buddhist sense has different roots and a slightly different meaning than the traditional English term. The Pāli word *karuna,* which we regularly translate as "compassion," never implied suffering. In fact, karuna itself is meant to be a tool to help overcome suffering. Bhikkhu Anālayo drives this point home with discussion of a Madhyama Āgama Sutra, which translates thus:

> Suppose a person comes and, standing to one side, sees that this traveler on an extended journey along a long road has become sick halfway, is exhausted and suffering extremely. He is alone and without a companion. The village behind is far away and he has not yet reached the village ahead. [The second person thinks,] "If he were to get an attendant, emerge from being in the wilderness far away and reach a village or town, and were to be given excellent medicine and be fed with nourishing and delicious food, be well cared for, then in this way this person's sickness would certainly subside." So that

person has extremely compassionate, sympathetic, and kind thoughts in the mind toward this sick person.[14]

Anālayo uses this passage to demonstrate a few significant points about the meaning of compassion, in this specifically Buddhist sense. It does not arise simply from seeing another suffering but is the *concern for their well-being*. More specifically, the concern for them to be free from suffering. As Anālayo states,

> Drawing a clear distinction between the realization that others are suffering and the wish for them to be free from suffering is important, since mentally dwelling on the actual suffering would be contemplation of *dukkha* [i.e., suffering itself] . . . in this way, the mind takes the vision of freedom from affliction as its object. Such an object can generate a positive, at times even a joyful state of mind, instead of resulting in sadness. [Thus] compassion does not mean to commiserate to the extent of suffering along with the other.[15]

Anālayo continues by pointing out how later texts explicitly state that commiserating with another's suffering is the "near enemy" of compassion. Cruelty is described as the "far enemy" of compassion. Thus, cruelty negates compassion and vice versa. But we must also be wary of commiseration, for this too can impede the development of true compassion in the Buddhist sense. In other words, commiseration impedes upon a type of compassion that can be mutually beneficial on the path toward freedom from suffering.

Psychological research on compassion and empathy tends to back up the value of such views, especially in terms of one's own sustainable capacity to care for others.

Types of Empathy and Compassion

Paul Bloom wrote in *Against Empathy: The Case for Rational Compassion* that "Empathy's narrow focus, specificity, and innumeracy mean that it's always going to be influenced by what captures our attention, by racial preferences, and so on. . . . Empathy will have to yield to reason if humanity is to have a future." However, Jamil Zaki emphasized the interplay between thought and emotions, along with empathy's role within such interplay. He calls this "psychological tuning." By changing our thoughts, we can adjust our feelings and ultimately the habits of those feelings and emotional reactions.[16] This is reminiscent of Candace Pert's biological research, described above.

In his book *The War for Kindness: Building Empathy in a Fractured World,* Zaki points out three distinct ways the word *empathy* is used and the human responses associated with them: sharing, thinking about, and caring about. "Sharing" is the basest level and often occurs almost immediately when seeing another's reaction. This is when you vicariously take on the emotions, moods, joys, or distress of another. We begin doing this as babies early on in life and see it on many levels of reactions as life continues on. For example, cognitive scientists observe how our neurons mirror the firing of those who react nearby us. The second category, "thinking about," refers to the more cognitive and imaginative level of empathy. When you see or hear about something that happens to another, you might picture that experience in your own mind, thinking about it from their perspective. The third, "caring about," refers to the actual concern and a wish or hope for another's suffering to diminish. Researchers call this "empathic concern," and it often comes with motivation to act in some way to help the other.

We may experience all three of these aspects of empathy when reacting to another, or only one of them; they do not necessarily come together. Many doctors experience caring while trying to block out the sharing aspects of empathy. Psychopaths typically clearly imagine what others are feeling (the cognitive aspect) without sharing or caring about those feelings. Those with autism tend to be on the opposite end of the spectrum; they may care very deeply about another's emotions, but struggle mentalizing them, imagining from the other's perspective.[17]

Zaki also noted that Buddhism encourages a form of compassion that does not entail taking on others' pain. He takes the same perspective as Anālayo in interpreting Buddhism's position that, whereas compassionate concern has benefits both to others and one's own psyche, commiseration is a potentially unhealthy form of compassion. Eve Ekman asserted the importance of this distinction: "If it goes too far one way it's 'that person, not my problem,' and if it doesn't happen, we can overidentify with the suffering around us."[18] Psychologists describe a similar distinction between empathetic distress and empathetic concern. Empathetic distress refers to

> feeling *as* someone else does by vicariously taking on their pain. Concern instead entails feelings *for* someone and wanting to improve their well-being. Concern and distress can seem like two sides of the same coin—if someone

else's pain hurts you, you have every reason to help them feel better—but they need not travel together. They are only weakly related: someone who experiences deep distress does not necessarily feel deep concern, and vice versa . . . in caring professions, knowing the difference between these states is vital. Distress motivates people to escape others' suffering, but caregivers can't do that without abandoning their post. This leaves them with a punishing psychological burden. In fact, of the different kinds of empathy, only distress tracks burnout among doctors, nurses, and social workers. Concern, on the other hand, gives them a way to emotionally connect with patients without taking on their pain, and caregivers who tend toward concern rather than distress are *less* likely to suffer from empathic injuries. In other words, empathy doesn't have to produce burnout at all, and experiencing the right kind might actually prevent it.[19]

Buddhist Compassion Practice and Meditation

Compassion, in the Buddhist sense, closely resembles empathic concern and is a skill emphasized for development widely across Buddhist schools and traditions. But compassion is not simply a skill that appears on its own. It is one of four *brahmavihāras,* alongside loving-kindness, sympathetic joy, and equanimity. Whether we carry compassion or sympathetic joy in our hearts depends upon the person in front of us. If they are suffering, we have compassion toward them, and if they are happy, we share in their joy. While with people in crisis, the two sides of this coin can sometimes flip back and forth quickly, or there can be multiple complex emotions piled on top of each other. Balancing the reflection of another's mental states with our own can be a challenging but worthwhile practice. Within the set of brahmavihāras, compassion is meant to be cultivated alongside loving-kindness and equanimity. We combine compassionate concern for another's well-being with loving-kindness toward them and a mental balance toward the situation at hand. Combining compassion with equanimity can be particularly important to help prevent compassion fatigue. The equanimity helps prevent us from becoming too attached toward the results of the situation in front of us.

Mahāyāna Buddhist schools compare compassion and wisdom to the two wings of a bird or other analogies that show how both are necessary for good action in the world. Chan master Venerable Hsing Yun sates, "only when compassion is mixed with *prajna* [wisdom], will it help others do good. . . . Compassion is like our two legs that make us mobile, and prajna is like our two eyes that help us tell the true from the false."[20]

Balancing the proper states of compassion with these various complementary qualities is not something that appears naturally at will. It requires practice; ideally, repeated and regular practice. Not only in situations with others, but through reflection and meditation on one's own as well. Buddhist traditions offer hundreds of activities for such development. For example, Kunga Lekpai Rinchen's fifteenth-century commentary "A Concise Guide to 'Parting from the Four Clingings'" lists several practices and subpractices to cultivate compassion, including thinking of all beings as one's own mother. He describes visualizing one's mother's suffering and strengthening the drive to free her from that suffering, before gradually spreading that mental state toward all sentient beings.[21]

The chapters that follow offer numerous other exercises to cultivate compassion and other states useful in crisis care. Rather than enter into the specifics here, however, it is important to cover some general issues in the application of Buddhist meditation and mindfulness practices.

Not all Buddhists meditate and not all Buddhist traditions espouse it, but various meditation practices are certainly common among many Buddhist schools, and many of the authors apply practices from their own traditions in the chapters that follow. Meditation is a word with very broad meaning, especially when describing Buddhist practices. The various languages and traditions include hundreds of words describing specific practices that often simply get translated to "meditation" in English. One broad term in Pāli encompassing most such practices is the word *bhavana,* literally meaning "cultivation of the mind and heart." It is with this word in mind that I use the word *meditation* in reference to the range of Buddhist practices.

Application of Buddhist meditation practices in secular situations has a growing yet complex recent history. Especially since Jon Kabat-Zinn and his promotion of Mindfulness Based Stress-Reduction (MBSR), there has been a steady growth of organizations, studies, and professionals using originally Buddhist practices in new secular applications. You don't need to look far to see one study or another purporting the benefits of mindfulness. While I don't want to take anything away from those developments, this movement should be contextualized in a few important ways before talking about their relevance for crisis care and within this volume.

A more recent pushback produced a number of valid critiques from different directions. Mindfulness is not for everyone and can sometimes lead to negative experiences as well. Willoughby Britton has been at the forefront of this growing piece of dialogue within the psychological sphere for over a decade and pointed out numerous dangers to be aware of, especially for those participating in lengthy retreats. In Buddhism, however, this is not a new discussion. Meditation can come with extreme challenges, and adverse side effects have been discussed in texts and warned by teachers for many centuries. This is precisely why many Buddhist meditation traditions warn that deeper practices should be done with an experienced teacher who can help individuals navigate such difficulties if and when they arise.

Another critique is that many scientific studies have very loose definitions of the "mindfulness" or "meditation" they are studying. For example, the U.S. Department of Health and Human Services conducted a study of over eight hundred mindfulness studies and found that due to the lack of clear conceptual or definitional understanding, the studies were actually "beset with uncertainty."[22]

Taking practices out of their originally complex textual and traditional contexts, the frameworks were shown to be *too* loose. When given relatively few instructions, it is natural that people let their minds move in a wide variety of ways as they try to meditate. As time goes on, scientists seem to be working to rectify this issue of defining the particular practice they are studying, but in terms of scientific understanding, we should recognize the infancy in which that field remains, and how many different types of mindfulness there really are. Studying one form of mindfulness and its effect on a particular condition means little for other types of mindfulness and its effects on that same condition.

A different critique skillfully elucidated by Funie Hsu, among others, points out that the secular mindfulness movement tends to erase Asian contributions through its focus on Kabat-Zinn and other white Western teachers. As she asserts, "secular mindfulness requires an ideology of white conquest that makes invisible the enduring efforts of Asian and Asian American Buddhists in maintaining the legacy of mindfulness practices."[23] Earlier Buddhists in the United

States were imprisoned, publicly ridiculed, placed in concentration camps, had their sacred texts burned, and toiled to change policies that led to that suffering. Those of us practicing today stand on the shoulders of their suffering and their efforts to bring these practices into the public eye. Hsu also links the erasure to "neoliberalism's sleight of invisible hand," showing how it is regularly linked to social and economic gains.

This relates to another significant issue, in that the secularization trend of mindfulness often takes away the ethical practices that traditionally came part and parcel with any contemplative practice. Right Mindfulness and Right Concentration are only two parts of the Noble Eightfold Path. Wisdom cannot be separated from virtue on the Buddhist path. These are fundamental tenets across schools for good reason. There has long been recognition that only being mindful about something does not necessarily come alongside morally benevolent action; it does not automatically lead to an end of suffering. If anything, the secular mindfulness movement has proven this point. Businesses use mindfulness programs not only as a way to keep worker stress lower, but to reduce turnover and avoid paying fair wages in the process. Mindfulness programs can be adapted by the military or businesses with questionable ethical practices to help dilute people's ethical misgivings about their participation. Just because we are mindful of our actions does not mean we act virtuously while doing it. Conversely, mindfulness detached from ethics and virtue can lead to furthering oppressive systems.

In Buddhism, Right Mindfulness and Right Concentration are meant to be practiced along with Right Effort, Right Thought, Right Speech, Right Action, and Right Livelihood. They are meant to be practiced in concert with the *discernment* of Right View. This requires that we follow the Four Noble Truths not only as a philosophical idea but as daily practice. We observe and comprehend suffering (the first truth). In doing so, we come to understand the roots or origins of that suffering and let it go or do what else we can to detangle ourselves from its grasp (second truth). This leads to realization of our release, at which point we reflect on and learn from the process (third truth). This allows us to walk the path anew with fresh and deeper awareness (fourth truth). Practiced consistently, it leads to a positive feedback loop of ever deepening awareness of suffering and release from it. This is the Four Noble Truths of which Buddhist meditation traditions are a part.

There is not one single type of mindfulness in Buddhism, much less one single path of practice. The paths are many and varied. There is often a phrase in Buddhist traditions referring to eighty-four thousand methods or ways to awakening. This reflects the view of many different ways for each of us to practice depending on what is right for each individual. There is not a set "one size fits all" structure. Some Buddhist traditions stick to one or a few particular practices, while others organically or systematically shift between numerous practices. The Thai Forest tradition, for example, uses many methods based on the Pāli canon (Nikāya) suttas. The method of choosing and adjusting practice in that tradition is reminiscent of Candace Pert's sailboat analogy mentioned above in "Fight, Flight . . . or Flourish." You adjust your practice and style depending on the conditions of the mind. A more apt and commonly referenced canonical analogy might be adjusting the tune and beat of your instrument to fit in the flow of a band or orchestra. Thānissaro Bhikkhu summarizes such sutras, saying:

> The comparison between music and meditation highlights a number of practical points in the development of meditative skill. First, it underscores the need for flexibility and ingenuity in the practice, tempered by an awareness of the limits of how far that flexibility can go. A skilled musician in the Buddha's time had to master not one but many tuning systems so as to handle a full range of musical themes, while simultaneously knowing which ways of tuning were unworkable. In the same way, a skilled meditator should know of many valid ways of tuning the mind to the theme of its meditation—and should have a command of them all so as to deal with various contingencies as they arise.[24]

Properly reflecting the diversity of traditions and practices can also open up more doors to the real possibilities of their application in society, including the ways those practices might relate to care.

I believe the chapters gathered in this volume present a great response to the above critiques and help present Buddhist practices that may be applicable to various needs of crisis care. The variety of practices mentioned within this volume are presented within the contexts of the specific schools and cultures where they originated, honoring the teachers and history that came before. There is no pretense about any one practice being a panacea, effective in all situations. Showing this diverse range of practices and traditions also helps show what variety there really is available and the different specific needs they have the potential to meet.

Whether applying practices, values, theories, or other aspects of Buddhist wisdom, the chapters that follow present a range of ways to deal with many aspects of crises and crisis care.

Chapter Outline

This volume's diverse authorship originated in more than ten different countries and come from at least twelve different Buddhist traditions, while each present their wisdom from various fields and perspectives in dealing with crisis. The chapters are separated into four parts. It should be mentioned that the issues in each of these chapters are complex and multifaceted; many of them could have been placed in more than one section and their themes are deeply interwoven. The order of placement simply provides some means to help navigate those complexities. However, the chapters of the book may be read in nearly any order depending on the relevance you find in the moment. They offer a variety of styles and approaches, depending on each author's experience and background.

The first section examines care during large-scale crises and disasters that stretch across a community, region, or the entire world. The second section borrows its title from three of the universal forms of suffering the Buddha described. It looks at crisis on a more personal level and care for those undergoing issues related to serious illness, aging, and dying. The third is a section focuses on caring for the care providers themselves. As mentioned above, compassion fatigue and related issues are common within caring professions and providing this meta level of care along with self-care are all the more important for those of us helping others through a crisis. Finally, there is a section on programs in different areas of the world created to train chaplains and others in the tools necessary to provide deeper levels of care.

The first section is the largest and begins with Reverend Dr. Victor Gabriel's chapter on a bodhisattva ecology. Bodhisattvas are beings who commit themselves to saving all living beings from suffering and wait to enter final nirvana until this goal is complete. In these times of global warming and increasingly common natural disasters, Gabriel utilizes the teachings of Sōtō Zen founder Dōgen and Shingon founder Kūkai. He relates them to Arne Næss's philosophy of deep ecology to propose a bodhisattva version of deep ecology to guide our lives during this period of planetary environmental crises. Dawn Neal's following chapter is from the perspective of community chaplaincy. She speaks to the overlapping crises of COVID-19, the California fires, and political agitation that were combining to fray nerves and create discord in her surrounding community. She promoted principles of listening and communication from chaplaincy as a form of public education while advocating for both-and solutions that listen to the diverse needs of communities. She also offers a model of social interaction and interdependence for those willing to be proactive in building community bridges. Following this, Vimalasara (Valerie Mason-John) addresses COVID, racial oppression, and other crises through the lens of the Four Noble Truths. She uses her background in addiction counseling and thirty-three years of Dharma practice to skillfully outline how, while some forms of pain may be beyond our control, these noble truths offer us a path through the "second dart" of suffering, namely the hatred, craving, and ignorance. Next, Hojin (Hye Sung) Park offers an essay on the role of Won Buddhist practice for immigrants and second-generation citizens struggling with identities within U.S. culture. Identity crises are not uncommon for those who have moved to a new culture and country, or their children, who deal with different cultures and languages when leaving and returning home. Park details these issues while also showing the role Won Buddhist meditation plays in helping people through such struggles, including finding their sense of identity.

Hitoshi Jin, in next chapter, reflects on his work during the devastating aftermath the 2011 Triple Disaster had on the people of northeastern Japan with the combined earthquake, tsunami, and nuclear disaster. He describes Buddhist disaster care during the immediate aftermath, when temples housed displaced survivors, and many volunteers gathered to offer trauma care and other forms of support. The chapter then shifts to describe how Jin helped establish emergency training services for volunteers so that they could properly care for the psychological needs of the people they encountered. The chapter also proposes a bodhisattva ideal for Buddhists in disaster and trauma care and introduces some of the related activities that the organization Zenseikyo has developed in the past decade. After this, my own chapter focuses on the work of Kaneta Taiō, mentioned at the beginning of this chapter, and the Café de Monk movement he initiated. I describe the principles of this café-style post-disaster care, outline Taiō's philosophy of care, and describe the masterful way in which he weaves music, humor, and activities into a holistic care experience for survivors during their times of deepest need. The author of the seventh chapter in this opening section, Chun Fai (Jeffrey) Ng, was a graduate student of Buddhist counseling in Hong Kong during the course of many of the protests and conflicts occurring in his city during 2019 and 2020. Ng writes about the mental health of the city as a whole before analyzing it through the lens of the Saṃdhinirmocana Sutra, a Yogācāra Buddhist text. He then proposes mental exercises and provides insights for personal well-being that he hopes can ultimately impact broader society as well. This section concludes with Dr. g, who combines poetry and prose to express the historical and modern oppression of Black people as well as a path to liberation. Doc weaves nonbinary Caribbean experience and wisdom from years as a clinical psychologist and Dharma teacher into lessons on three doors of liberation: emptiness, signlessness, and aimlessness.

The second area this book explores is bedside care for individuals dealing with personal crises related to aging, illness, and death. In the first chapter of this section, Manling Lim, who served as a chaplain within a hospital's Level I trauma center, offers a personal account of her experience being called to assist the distressed fiancée of a patient in cardiopulmonary arrest, a medical emergency referred to as "code blue" in hospitals. The chapter details her internal struggles and achievements during the encounter as well as the methods used to help her calm the fiancée, including prayer, a contemplative finger labyrinth, and breathing guidance. Anna Gagnon provides, in the following chapter, a hospital chaplain's wisdom on constructing ritual and prayer for patients in crisis. She provides examples from her experience and describes her process of speaking from the heart and carefully listening to patients' needs to weave together the right words for each individual. Next, Noel Alumit connects his award-winning writing career with his chaplaincy training to describe his very personal experience of discovering his brain aneurysm. He relies particularly upon the story of the Buddha and Kisa Gotami in helping himself come to terms with the condition and find a sense of restoration. Kin Cheung (George) Lee's chapter then discusses talking to people with cancer, especially those who've been recently diagnosed. He explores this especially through his work with the "Note, Know, Choose" model, a Buddhist counseling approach he developed.

The earlier chapters in this section touch on themes of serious illness and disease, but the latter chapters of the section discuss those who face the aging and dying process. A medical technician originally from Indonesia, Dian (Dee) Sutawijaya describes her hospice work and the trials her patients face during the onset of dementia and at their very final stages of life. She finds inspiration in the Anāthapiṇḍika Sutra and its description of Sāriputta's own deathbed care, while providing case studies of her work and how she adapts her Buddhist-inspired care to provide for the needs of Christian patients. Finally, Lourdes Argüelles (Lopon Dorje Khandro) shares her wisdom from years of experience in counseling traumatized refugees at the U.S.-Mexico border. Through extended dialogue and the practices of Tonglen and the deity Amitābha as well as prayers and offerings to Mexican saints, Argüelles shares how she came to incorporate Tibetan Buddhist and Mexican folk Catholic practices into her care through a case study of Emilio, a young man with AIDS. Argüelles and Emilio jointly developed a series of practices that helped Emilio peacefully navigate his dying process and Argüelles to broaden and integrate her charnel ground experiences into her everyday life.

The third section of this volume brings the focus back to care providers themselves, looking at issues and methods of caring for distressed or exhausted staff and self-care. The first chapter by Shushin R. A. Peterson compares the work of chaplaincy to a Zen koan titled the "Case of Master Ma" from the *Blue Cliff Record*. Peterson uses this story, Master Ma's response, traditional commentaries, and teachings on Buddha Nature to show how those providing care can more skillfully provide presence and ask clarifying questions to those in need. The next three chapters look particularly at different situations and methods to care for the needs of hospital staff, but provide methods that are very applicable to a range of other caregivers. Acala Xiaoxi Wang tells a story, adapted from her own experience, of a night and day in the life of an ICU chaplain, while tasked with not just working through the night but ministering to staff care with a group support activity the next morning. After discussing her internal struggles and initial consternation about the request, Wang outlines the path she followed in order to design and implement an activity that could bring relief, cohesion, and healing to the team of employees. Stephanie Barnes (Repa Nyima Ozer) then brings both her Tibetan Buddhist background and chaplaincy experience to the fore with a case study explaining how she helped integrate her tradition's mandala practice into daily contemplations that ICU staff could readily use for self-care and in cultivating compassion within a

medical ICU. She adapted the various visualizations and mantras into a nondenominational secularized form of practice that fit the space of the ICU so that
staff could embody the practices as they walked through the building. Following this, Shushin Peterson shares the Stress-management Mindfulness Series
he helped establish during the COVID response at a hospital where he was
working to help care for overworked hospital staff. He shares what he included
for these Buddhist-inspired yet secularized and open sessions. The chapter compares more Buddhist-inspired and secularized forms of mindfulness and ana-
lyzes how this model might be adapted and shared within other similar settings
in the future.

In the next chapter, Chenxing Han provides a vivid and chaotic scene from
her hospital residency as a case study to show the importance of accepting care
as a chaplain or caregiver. She beautifully interlaces her story with poetry from
the Cambodian Dharma song tradition to help drive the points home. Finally,
Alex Baskin discusses the value of play for self-care. He frames the discussion
around the struggles and stress of individuals during the COVID pandemic
and systemic race issues. He describes the activities of InterPlay, an organization which facilitates mindful embodied movement, to exemplify a way to
release various pressures, increase resiliency, and prevent burnout.

The final section of the volume focuses more on the training of care providers. How do we best train people to care for others who are going through times
of deep need in their lives? Taniyama Yōzō is a Pure Land Buddhist priest who
previously served as one of Japan's first Buddhist hospice chaplains and helped
found Japan's first interfaith chaplaincy certification program in the wake of
the 2011 disaster. In this chapter he discusses the precursor to that program,
the "Heart Consultation Room." Taniyama details the development of the
center, various forms of care they provided to survivors, and some of the issues
in adapting Western spiritual care to Japanese culture. Wang Fengshuo's chapter then discusses how the aging population in China is creating severe issues
due to the lack of people and institutions to care for all the elderly needs. In
response, Shanghai's Jade Buddha Temple launched a revolutionary Life Education College in 2020 to train individuals in Buddhist-inspired end-of-life care
practices. In this chapter, the program's founder introduces the background of
hospice in Shanghai and China, the issues they encountered while creating such

a new Buddhist program in China, and the extra challenges 2020 brought to a nascent program.

Following this, four experienced Buddhist chaplaincy instructors (Jitsujo T. Gauthier, Daijaku Kinst, Leigh Miller, and Elaine Yuen) collaborate to describe the process and stages of chaplaincy training in the United States. For those interested in taking a deeper look into how they might help others in crisis or suffering in other ways, this chapter can help show the steps you might follow to undertake one such path of training. It is also a process influential upon many other world chaplaincy training systems. In the final chapter, Leigh Miller, the Director of Academic Programs at Maitripa College, offers a look into the training of chaplains and others in spiritual care through their graduate school and MDiv program. This chapter builds on the previous one by showing more depth in how a Buddhist tradition influences such training in care. It also includes interviews of graduates regarding how they are putting that training into practice in the field, being with those in crisis, and what their different Buddhist backgrounds mean for them in this field.

Through this thorough and diverse look into what Buddhists contribute to crisis care, we hope that readers might bring away many ideas that can inspire and be further adapted in helping people and communities during periods of deep need. May any merits gained from these efforts be dedicated to sentient beings' release from suffering in this world.

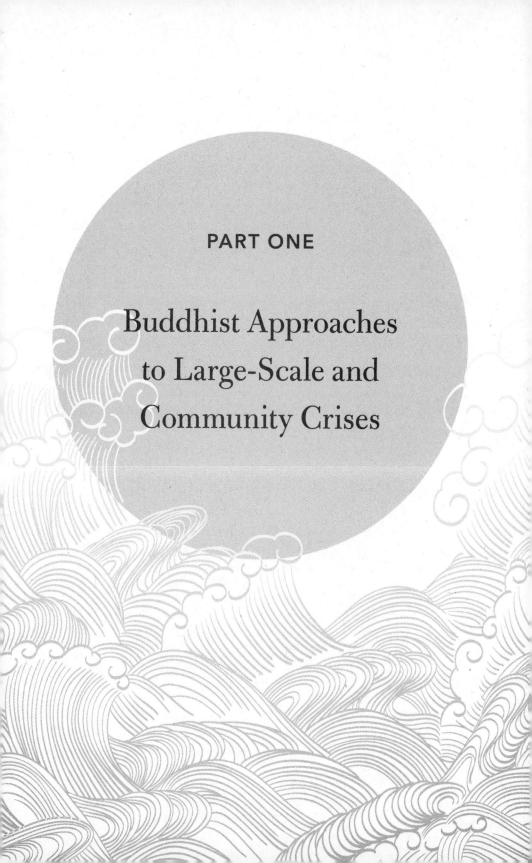

PART ONE

Buddhist Approaches to Large-Scale and Community Crises

1

THE ECOLOGY OF
THE BODHISATTVA

Victor Gabriel

Sentient beings are numberless; I vow to save them.
Consuming desires are endless; I vow to stop them.
Bio-relations are intricate; I vow to honor them.
Nature's way is beautiful; I vow to become it.[1]

Introduction

Today, the extent of our environmental crisis is beyond our imagination. Governments have failed to demonstrate consistent intent and ability to address the multidimensional nature of our environmental problems. Ecology is the study of the relationship between organisms and their environment. I would like to propose an ecological movement that draws from both deep ecology and the bodhisattvas' purification of the buddha-field[2] or, in other words, a "buddha-ecology." In doing so, I hope to explicate and extend our understanding of buddha-field by drawing upon the work of Kūkai (774–835) and Dōgen (1200–1253), two of history's most famous Japanese Buddhist teachers. Deep ecology is an ecology movement that has gone beyond the presupposition that humans are the stewards of creation or nature and the peak of the hierarchal pyramid of evolution. Instead, the movement suggests that we inter-be with nature as equal partners. This new vision of the ecology can benefit from an understanding of the bodhisattvas' purification of the buddha-ecology. In the Mahāyāna Buddhist tradition, bodhisattvas are those who are intent on enlightenment, but forgo the final steps until they have compassionately acted to save all other sentient beings from suffering. We will broaden this definition by envisioning bodhisattvas as those who have decided to move beyond the boundaries of their ego to remembering their interdependence with the buddha-ecology. This process of remembering is the purification of the buddha-ecology. It takes place at both an absolute and relative level. We will begin with the historical roots of the deep ecology movement and its perspective or view. After that we will explore the view of Buddhist ecology.

The Historical Roots of Deep Ecology

The deep ecology movement developed from the ecological revolution of 1960s.[3] The ecological revolution began with the publication in 1962 of Rachel Carson's *Silent Spring*. Carson questioned the then prevailing anthropocentric view of Western culture that humans had the innate right to dominate and manage nature. Instead, she advocated an ecology that saw humans as part of the biointegrity of nature.

In 1966, at a meeting of the American Association for the Advancement of Science, medieval historian Lynn White presented a paper titled "The Historical Roots of Our Ecological Crisis," in which he strongly reinforced Carson's view. White suggested that Western Christianity sought to understand God's mind by discovering how creation works while Eastern Christianity continued to perceive nature as a symbolic system through which God speaks to humankind. Thus, Western Christianity has led to an anthropocentric worldview that placed humans above and beyond nature and encouraged its exploitation. It was his opinion that Western Christianity bears a huge burden of guilt[4] for the ecological problems of the day. He argued that "since the roots of our trouble are so largely religious, the remedy must also be essentially religious, whether we call it that or not."[5] White proposed as a solution from within Western Christianity—the paradigm of Francis of Assisi who believed in the "equality of all creatures, including man (sic)," and "a democracy of all God's creatures."[6] As we will see below, this nonanthropic position can be found in the concept of bodhisattvas' purification of the buddha-ecology. This idea initiated the ecological revolution, which, unlike previous conservation movements, sought not only to promote ecology as beneficial to all species but also to clash with power centers that were in favor of "gratuitous development."[7]

About the same time, Arne Næss (1912–2009), a Norwegian philosopher, began studying the interaction between philosophy and ecology. In 1972, at the Third World Futures conference in Bucharest, Romania, Næss differentiated between deep and shallow ecology, and this marked the birth of the deep ecology movement. Næss continued to refine the position of deep ecology, and presently we have three main characterizations of deep ecology.[8] However, our discussion will focus only on broader philosophical positions as found in the Deep Ecology Platform. This new philosophical comprehension unfortunately comes with intensification of our ecological crisis.[9]

The View of Deep Ecology: The Deep Ecology Platform

In his 1972 Bucharest paper, Næss defines shallow ecology as being concerned with pollution, resource depletion, and human well-being as distinct from the rest of nature.[10] On the other hand, the Deep Ecology Platform articulates the concerns of deep ecology.[11] There are eight points in this platform:

1. The well-being and flourishing of all organisms, including humans, have value in themselves. This value is unrelated to the utility of the nonhuman world to human purposes.

    This is the standpoint of ecocentrism. Some deep ecologists, as in the 1972 Bucharest paper, have taken the stronger position of ecospherical egalitarianism, where every organism has an innate right to live and prosper—not just an intrinsic value but intrinsic right. An anthropocentric position where we have alienated ourselves from nature and have adopted a master-slave relationship with nature has only resulted in our alienation from and with ourselves (since we have always been part of nature).

2. Richness and diversity of life forms contribute to the fulfillment of these values and are values in themselves. Diversity increases the potential for survival, for new modes of life, and for the richness of life. Shallow ecological perceptions like the "struggle for life" and the "survival of the

fittest" need to be reconsidered through the lens of coexistence and cooperation in complex eco-relationships.

3. Humans have no right to reduce this richness and diversity of life except to satisfy critical needs.

4. The flourishing of human life and cultures is congruent with a smaller human population. The flourishing of nonhuman life requires a smaller human population.

5. Present human interference with the nonhuman world is excessive and the situation is speedily deteriorating. All organisms, including humans, have modified their ecosystems, but humans need to reconsider the nature and extent of their interference to their ecosystems. Most of the wilderness preserved outside of human interference is too small to allow for evolutionary speciation of nonhuman life forms.

6. The policies that affect basic economic, technological, and ideological structures must change. The resulting state of affairs will consequently be different from the present. Economic growth based on the cycle of consumption is incongruent with points 1 to 5. New structures must arise from a deep interaction with the local ecosystems at a grassroots level.

7. This ideological change will come from appreciating the quality of life rather than an emphasis on increasing standards of living.

8. Those who subscribe to the previous points have an obligation to indirectly or directly implement changes.

The View of Buddhist Ecology: Nature of Nature

Buddhist ecology offers another perspective beyond the duality of anthropocentrism and ecocentrism and whether human interests will ever be adequately considered in ecocentrism. There is a vast body of Buddhist literature that expresses Buddhism's relationship to nature, and this immensity has sometimes led to its perspective being obscured. In *Dharma Rain,* Stephanie Kaza and Kenneth Kraft have found three themes that articulate the "View" of Buddhist ecology.[12] These three themes are: a reverence for life, nature as teacher and refuge, and the nature of nature.[13]

The nature of nature in its absolute aspect is *śūnyatā* or emptiness. This emptiness is an emptiness of labeling, permanence, and independence. It does not mean a nihilistic vacuum, but rather the presence of nonreferent interdependence. This nonreferent interdependence is the buddha-field or buddha-ecology. This interdependence is embodied in all phenomena, including our ecosphere. Thich Nhat Hanh explains this interdependence with this metaphor:

> In one sheet of paper, you can see the sun, the clouds, the forest, and even the logger. The paper is made of nonpaper elements. The entire world conspired to create it and it exists within it. . . . Breathing out, we realize that the atmosphere is made of all of us. I am, therefore you are. You are, therefore I am. We inter-are.[14]

This buddha-ecology is pure because it transcends the duality of permanence and impermanence, the duality of beauty and ugliness, the duality of bliss and sorrow, and the duality of self and no-self.[15] To experience the purity of the buddha-ecology is to experience the beauty of this interdependence. In Robert Thurman's *The Holy Teaching of Vimalakīrti*, the magnificence of the buddha-ecology is expressed by way of metaphor in the miracle where the Buddha reveals the true nature of nature: "Thereupon the Lord touched the ground of this billion-world-galactic universe with his big toe, and suddenly it was transformed into a huge mass of precious jewels, a magnificent array of many hundreds of thousands of clusters of precious gems."[16] *The Holy Teaching of Vimalakīrti* goes on to explain that the reason beings do not experience "the splendid display of virtues of the buddha-field of the Tathāgata is due to their own ignorance" and that beings "see the splendor of the virtues of the buddha-fields of the Buddhas according to their own degree of purity."[17]

Kūkai, in the *Meanings of Sound, Letter and Reality (Shō-ji-jisō gi)*, quotes the Avataṃsaka Sutra, saying, "the body of the Buddha is inconceivable / All worlds are contained within and on each of his hairs are manifested infinite worlds . . ."[18] He explains how the Buddha and his teachings pervade all the parts of our phenomenal world.

However, in accord with our various degrees of defilements, we envision various realities. Dōgen Zenji in verse 16 of the Mountains and Rivers Sutra describes how a single phenomenon—water—can be viewed and experienced differently by humans on the one hand and dragons and fish on the other:

> Now when dragons and fish see water as a palace, it is just like human beings seeing a palace. They do not think it flows. If an outsider tells them, "What you see as a palace is running water," the dragons and fish will be astonished, just as we are when we hear the words, "Mountains flow." Nevertheless, there may be some dragons and fish who understand that the columns and pillars of palaces and pavilions are flowing water.[19]

We should also bear in mind that our interdependence is not something far removed from us. The possibility of awareness is present in this very moment. In verse 21 of the Mountains and Rivers Sutra, Dōgen Zenji expresses this as, "Water is only the true thus-ness of water. Water is water's complete virtue; it is not flowing. When you investigate the flowing of a handful of water and the not-flowing of it, full mastery of all things is immediately present."[20] The transformation we make from our conventional perspective to the absolute view of interdependence exists as explained by *The Holy Teaching of Vimalakīrti*, "to bring about the maturity of inferior living beings."[21]

The Ethics of Deep Ecology and Buddha-Ecology

This brings us to the discussion on how we as eco-bodhisattvas can purify our buddha-ecology or ecosphere so that we and all beings can see the splendor of virtues of this buddha-ecology or ecosphere. Activism is the process of taking direct action to achieve a goal. Our goal here is the purification of the buddha-ecology. Unlike most social activism, our activism or engaged spiritual action involves changing not just social structures but also changing entire social paradigms. However, it is not a task fraught with fear and hope, for our ecosphere, with its environmental issues, is already the magnificent buddha-ecology. The activism is derived from a set of ethics or principles of right conduct. In both deep ecology and buddha-ecology, ethics and activism are interdependently related.

The Buddhist Precepts and Refuge

The ethics of the buddha-ecology are the Buddhist precepts.[22] Without precepts, the practice of buddha-ecology or of Buddhism, according to Robert Aitken, "tends to become a hobby, made to fit the needs of ego."[23] Aitken maintains that the core of all Buddhist precepts found in the various Buddhist traditions is the Refuge vows.[24] In Aitken's tradition, Japanese Zen, the refuge vows to the Buddha, Dharma, and Sangha are explained as going for refuge in realization, truth, and harmony. The goal of these vows is to make us harmonious with ourselves, with our community, and with reality: the buddha-ecology.

To be in harmony with the buddha-ecology is to be in touch with reality. Thich Nhat Hanh's introduction to the Fourteen Mindfulness Trainings of the Order of Interbeing offers an explanation of the words of the Vietnamese characters for interbeing, *tiep hien*.[25] *Tiep* refers to being in touch. Hanh suggests that precepts invite us to be in touch with reality, the reality of the mind and the reality of the world and buddha-ecology. To be in touch with the mind means to be aware of inner processes of the mind. To be in touch with reality means to be in touch with everything: the animal, vegetable, mineral, and energetic realms.

Among these Buddhist precepts are the bodhisattva vows. The bodhisattva vows are a means for us to be in harmony and in touch with the reality of the buddha-ecology. The bodhisattva vows offer us six pathways that can be taken simultaneously or gradually in order. The six pathways are the six *pāramitas* or six transcendent perfections: generosity, discipline, patience, joyful effort, meditation, and penetrating insight. They are not ordinary virtues, for these virtues are interdependent with emptiness. These virtues are in harmony or in touch with the buddha-ecology. This interdependent relationship between these transcendent perfections and emptiness is the experience of the transcendent perfection of penetrating insight. This experience is beyond language or concepts and yet can only be evoked through words.

In the transcendent perfection of generosity, we vow to extend ourselves beyond the territory of our ego into the expanse of the buddha-ecology. In

the *Guide to the Bodhisattvas' Way of Life (Bodhisattvacaryāvatāra)*, this is
expressed as follows:

> Thus for everything that lives,
> As far as are the limits of the sky,
> May I provide their livelihood and nourishment
> Until they pass beyond the bounds of suffering.[26]

In the transcendent perfection of discipline, we vow to recall again and again
our inseparability with the buddha-ecology. In the transcendent perfection
of patience, we vow to use even negative emotional states as reminders of
the buddha-ecology. In the transcendent perfection of joyous effort, we vow
to remember that at the absolute level we are inseparable from the buddha-
ecology. In the transcendent perfection of meditation, we vow to experience
buddha-ecology in every moment.

The ethics of the deep ecology and the bodhisattva precepts ensure that we
will be transformed when we act based on them. For the deep ecology movement to be interpenetrated by buddha-ecology, we need to use the Deep Ecology Platform and the six transcendent perfections. We recognize both the
absolute and relative level of our ecological crisis. These ecological issues do not
exist at the absolute level, but they do exist at a relative level. At the relative level,
we are invited to engage in activism and solutions. These solutions can be found
in Part 5 of *A Buddhist Response to the Climate Emergency*, which include: using
wind power; solar-thermoelectric power; solar photovoltaic power; tidal power;
geothermal power; ending energy waste; ending the use of the internal combus-
tion engine; drawing down carbon with biochar; reducing the carbon footprint
of the meat industry; ending deforestation; and engaging in reforestation.[27] Of
course, these solutions need to be improved, and this is another area of bodhisattva activity.

Conclusion

Joanna Macy calls the above processes the "greening of self."[28] She notes three
trends regarding why this greening of self will become a reality for us. First,
the small ego-self is threatened by the ecological problems we are facing.[29]
These ecological problems threaten our future certainty, and the ego-self needs

certainty. Secondly, what she calls "new paradigm sciences" see life as organized systems that are sustained in and by their relationships. Thirdly is the popularity of nondualistic spiritualities like Buddhism, which advocate an interdependent relationship with our environment. She suggests that as ecological issues are not widely discussed, the greening of self will be crucial, "because there is nothing more preoccupying or energy-draining than that which we repress."[30]

The greening of self leads to the eco-self. This is the "self" that is interdependent with the environment. I would like to suggest that the eco-self is the bodhisattva who has realized their interdependence with the buddha-ecology, who has purified the buddha-ecology. In realizing the purity of the buddha-ecology, we realize the inseparability of environmental issues and the purity of the buddha-ecology, the inseparability of appearance and emptiness. When we purify our conventional or imaginary reality, we end up with the relative world in its nonconceptual purity. This purity, being nonconceptual, is beyond expression. By being thoroughly processed by the ethics and activism of buddha-ecology, we come to this nonconceptual purity. At the same time, as the ethics and activism of buddha-ecology and we ourselves are inseparable from the purity of the buddha-ecology itself, we do *not* act so as to achieve the purity of the buddha-ecology. We act because we are inseparable from that purity.

Here, I showed how the concept of Buddha Nature and the deep ecology movement could inform each other. As Lynn White had argued, since the roots of the desecration of our ecosphere are largely religious, we need to find new spiritual ecological models that express our interdependence with our ecosphere. The View that is derived from the bodhisattva's purification of buddha-ecology offers us not only a refreshing way to view our ecological issues but also a new way to overcome these ecological issues. Our ecological ethics and activism must come from being in touch with and in harmony with our ecosphere or buddha-ecology. Our ecological ethics and activism are the conventional path we traverse to realize the purity of the buddha-ecology.

2

RESPONDING TO MULTIPLE CRISES AND THE ROLES OF COMMUNITY CHAPLAINCY

Dawn Neal

I n this chapter, I offer an example of one way that Buddhist chaplains and teachers might meet some of the crises unfolding in our societies today. I then introduce a broader context of how our Buddhist presence and voices can fit into larger community systems, a human and societal version of the kind of interdependence Victor Gabriel discussed in chapter 1.

The crisis referred to here is divisive polarization, which I believe deserves our careful attention and response. That said, my hope is that these words empower you to meet any social ill or crisis that *you* feel called to respond to. Each of us will respond to a crisis in our own unique way. Perhaps the perspective and process touched on here could be adapted by Buddhist chaplains, teachers, or others to address any number of social or environmental challenges.

In my case, I felt moved to respond to the increasingly divisive, at times inflammatory, rhetoric unfolding over local social media in the summer and autumn of 2020. I voiced my response through an invited guest perspective in a local paper. This and other opportunities for broader community engagement emerged through my participation in the Peninsula Solidarity Cohort, a group of forty spiritual and faith leaders working for compassion and justice in San Mateo County, California.[1]

Writing these guest columns has been an opportunity to speak, as a Buddhist teacher and chaplain, to the general public, many of whom are not necessarily familiar with Buddhist teachings. With that in mind, I wrote this essay, "Responding to Multiple Crises," in plain English. I emphasized real-world relatable examples while overtly and implicitly weaving in wisdom of some early Buddhist teachings from Theravāda Pāli texts:

Responding to Multiple Crises: A Call for a Community Ethic of Compassion[2]

San Mateo Daily Journal, *"Guest Perspective," June 4, 2020. Reprinted with permission.*

"All is burning," an ancient Buddhist wisdom teaching says. We scarcely need a reminder that intense fires around the Bay Area and across California sweep through our forested spaces, threatening or destroying communities in their path. Smoke strains our very breathing. Access to outdoor spaces, such vital outlets now, is constrained. All of this compounds pandemic-related uncertainty, stressors, and loss. In this sad and difficult time, some of us are losing apartments, mortgages, livelihoods, family members, or life itself. Many people feel anxious and agitated. Many of us feel threatened.

Feeling threatened generates fight-flight reactions that are critical when fleeing a burning structure. Unfortunately, the same fight-flight vigilance becomes a toxin to our health when chronically activated. Habitual fight-flight responses wind us up even as they wear us down. This happens when we are reacting to overlapping disasters, or reacting to the opportunistic voices of greed and hatred that seek to further inflame our fears and anger and irrevocably divide us.

Feeling threatened rarely evokes anyone's best behavior. It is far too easy to be swayed by reactive emotions that temporarily hijack our nervous systems, and thus also hijack our openness to other points of view, our generosity, and trust in our common humanity.

Neighbors, too many of our hearts and minds are burning. Our human biological reactions to perceived threats inflame many hearts with anger and hostility. The smoke of delusion can shrink our minds' capacities for reason. When our internal worlds, our values, hearts, minds, and senses are impacted this way, we are experiencing what the ancient teachings meant by "all is burning." In such reactive states, it's all too easy to habitually react with judgment, anger, words, and actions that burn through relationships, alienate families, dehumanize those who think differently, and wear thin the fabric of community itself.

We have other alternatives.

As a chaplain, I have often found that even strong anger, hostility, and fear from feeling threatened are instinctive attempts to protect a sense of vulnerability underneath. It's possible to see beneath our vigilance, meet our fear and vulnerability, and see that these feelings are based on deep caring: for each of us, at the most basic level, our life, the lives of our families, are the core of what we hold dear. What matters most.

For those who truly connect with the care for our own lives, it's possible to look around and realize that for nearly all persons, this care for their life is dear. Taken to heart, the resulting empathy and compassion reveal how important it is not to harm others by taking away what matters most to them. At a core level, people want to live with a basic sense of safety, health, and well-being. Whether black, brown, white, red, purple, or blue, we wish to live, to thrive, and be respected. To be treated fairly.

Realizing that this wish is common to each of us can open the door to respecting, even caring for, the lives of others. Lots of us are having a hard time right now. Sometimes we are wound up, nerves frayed, perhaps in fear, trauma, or worse. This is true for those we love, and true of those who think very differently than we do. We don't need to agree to feel a sense of compassion. We can agree to disagree and still help each other out. Neighbor to neighbor.

I am not advocating we paper over our differences. Instead, I am suggesting that we can, together, both contribute to a community ethic of compassion and engage in caring confrontation and constructive dialogue. We can prioritize public safety *and* act to end police brutality. We can advocate for racial justice *and* address our neighbors' fears of change. We can protest—and raise voices against protests—with restraint and respect.

We can call out—reject—hate speech and divisive rhetoric, regardless of our political party. We can channel the heat in our hearts toward constructive, compassionate action for the common good: getting out the vote, protecting the marginalized, ensuring the basic rights of citizenship in our democracy.

Finally, to the extent we can cool the fires in our own hearts, *and* be compassionately engaged with others when their hearts are inflamed, the more cohesion our community will have going forward to address the many problems we face. A community ethic of compassionate engagement strengthens our resilience to rebuild and recover together.

·

As many readers will likely have noticed, this short newspaper essay opened with a reference to the Buddha's famed Fire Sermon (Ādittapariyāya Sutta, Saṃyutta Nikāya 35.28). I used references to that teaching—which speaks of how lust, hatred, and delusion inflame our senses and minds—to highlight the danger of reactivity and hostility to our hearts, minds, and relationships.

Later, speaking from the perspective of a chaplain, I implicitly invoked another early Buddhist teaching, the Rājan Sutta (Udāna 5.1). In it the Buddha states that since we hold ourselves and our lives most dear, we should recognize that others hold their lives dear as well. With that in mind, "you shouldn't hurt others if you love yourself." Since self-love is by no means universally available in our culture, I couched this teaching in terms of the care readers feel for their lives and families, "what matters most." The call for compassionate engagement at the end of this pragmatic piece echoes the emphasis that all Buddhist traditions place on compassion and kindness.

This essay, as well as another written earlier in the pandemic, engaged an audience of people from different faiths, classes, political orientations, and walks of life. It is one small example of *community chaplaincy*, bringing the perspective of a Buddhist chaplain and teacher into a wider community forum.

Offering teachings, however, does not need to be a Buddhist's only means of action. As Buddhist spiritual care providers—chaplains or teachers—we support others through our practice, understanding, and presence. The form of that support is often a spiritual care conversation. Through deep listening, interpersonal mindfulness, and compassion, we follow the thread of a person's narrative and helped them connect to their inner resources. Indeed, although more commonly known as the term to refer to sacred Buddhist texts, the word *sutta* (Pāli) or *sūtra* (Sanskrit) can be translated as "narrative," "discourse," or "thread." In this next section, I introduce a model of how Buddhist leaders and others can help weave beneficial community narratives and cultivate ways of counteracting social ills exacerbated by crisis.

Buddhist Leaders Are Part of an Interdependent Societal System

I was reminded of the multiple meanings of *sutta* or *sūtra* when I attended a 2020 online depolarization summit. The summit was convened to address a growing trend of polarization, that is, sharply divisive adherence to extreme views.[3] While the summit addressed the United States, many panelists brought expertise from around the world, and brought their concern about the global rise of violent community polarization.

One panelist, Sadia Hameed, chose to focus on how a single thread, a simple narrative of "maintaining calm, accepting election results, and supporting a peaceful transition of power" could be beneficial to the community. She used this thread to model a "Whole of Society" response to Americans' deeply polarized election. The Whole of Society's Ecosystem Approach illustrated how different people and organizations can work in mutually reinforcing ways to support this peaceful narrative.[4]

Hameed pointed to the importance of influencers speaking to their own communities in their own language, supporting the narrative. Because she is part of a nongovernmental organization (NGO), her model featured an NGO as the central perspective, like the center of a flower. The petals around the flower were a cluster of overlapping community groups that included faith communities, educators, businesses, philanthropy, government agencies, and local news and media outlets. Someone modeling a simple narrative from another organization would likely start by putting theirs in the center.

Each group has its own interests, but through communication, they established common priorities. Influencers within each group could amplify beneficial narratives for all of these groups, in their own language. This created an emergent beneficial cycle, and as beneficial societal ideas gain traction in one community, they would often cross over to another. In this way, prosocial, beneficial ideas can mutually reinforce each other and the common priorities of all groups. From a Buddhist perspective, Ms. Hameed was modeling a practical, community-oriented example of interdependence and conditionality.

Hameed highlighted the role of faith communities as particularly important. I would add that this role increasingly includes nontraditional faith contexts (nontraditional, that is, for mainstream Americans). A growing percentage of Americans, for example, name that their primary—or only—contact with religious or spiritual guidance is outside traditional Western organized religion. Instead, spiritual guidance tends to be with chaplains or through attending activities in spiritual communities, such as yoga classes or meditation groups run by Buddhist teachers.

In short, Buddhist care providers and teachers, together with other religious and spiritual professionals, already function as important parts of a larger social ecosystem. By being aware of this, we have the opportunity to contribute more consciously to a whole ecology of people and organizations working toward a better society. Our presence, wisdom, and voices can help to weave a healthy and resilient counteracting response to the divisive forces in our communities. Whether our voices are heard one-on-one, in a group, or through writing, they can be beneficial prosocial contributions. As Buddhists, it is easy to recognize the wisdom of understanding beneficial community action through the lens of interdependence. Each part of the community ecosystem can contribute ways to ameliorate harmful societal trends, such as divisive polarization, and cultivate wholesome or healthy ones. Such contributions are a community version of the Four Great Efforts in Buddhist teachings, which encourage us to cultivate and maintain wholesome and healthy states while preventing and abandoning unhealthy ones.[5]

In Mahāyāna Buddhist practice and teachings, the kind of interdependence seen in this community ecosystem approach is sometimes described as "co-arisen" and "emergent." And, of course, some beneficial mutually reinforcing messages or actions organically emerge among, say, like-minded community members and organizations. This is a very good thing. The Whole of Society process, however, also emphasizes how intentionally forming connections and collaborations across different societal sectors increases opportunities for mutually reinforcing positive change.

From a Buddhist perspective, the Whole of Society model's ecosystem approach echoes not only a Mahāyāna understanding of interdependence and dependent arising, but also the early Buddhist principle of general conditionality, otherwise known as "this-that conditionality" (idappaccayatā).[6] The first half of this-that conditionality states, "When this exists, that comes to be; with the arising of this, that arises."[7] From this early Buddhist perspective, forming connections and relationships between different people and organizations across each community cultivates beneficial conditions for the future arising of mutually reinforcing positive action. In my own experience, such connections often form one conversation, one event, at a time.[8]

Organizations such as the local interfaith group I mentioned at the beginning of this chapter, Peninsula Solidarity Cohort, are well positioned to cultivate such beneficial conditions through conversations and building relationships. The interfaith cohort also coordinated and reinforced ways to support a peaceful narrative and transition of power. Because the cohort existed, the regular newspaper contributions came to be. Because we had dedicated time to interfaith dialogue, I could use my own language in a published column to support and reinforce priorities agreed on across many spiritual and faith communities: peaceful, meaningful discourse, and using voting as an expression of civic engagement.

Cultivating individual, local, and community relationships and connections fits in well with an overarching principle of depolarization: *Meaningful change starts locally, even hyperlocally.* Apparently, the kinds of changes required to depolarize nations are not effective if mandated from the top down. Rather, such changes emerge from specificity—interactions and collaborations like town halls, neighborhood discussions, and even individual conversations. In fact, several depolarization panelists highlighted something all practicing Buddhists understand: Meaningful change starts within our individual hearts and in minds, and ripples out through our speech and actions.

Buddhist teachers, leaders, and chaplains are well equipped to facilitate vital conversations to counteract crises, with individuals and in the broader community. The essay above offers only one small example of how Buddhists can act as a positive societal force, in concert with other well-intentioned people. There are many other possibilities.

We can inspire and echo the emergence of goodness in others around us organically, remembering that our efforts always exist within a larger context of concerned and caring community members and institutions. That said, to enact beneficial change it is also helpful to cultivate conditions, including relationships, that allow us to act in concert with other parts of the social ecosystem. Then, we can clearly see and contribute toward common and mutually beneficial purposes rather than being like the blind men of the famous Buddhist parable, only comprehending one part of the elephant in the room.[9]

3

CRISIS: THE SECOND DART OF SUFFERING

Vimalasara (Valerie Mason-John)

As a Buddhist practitioner I continue to learn and think of challenging life events as a constant flow of this miraculous world, rather than a crisis. If I am to name one thing in the Dharma that has schooled me during the past thirty-three years, it has been that nothing is certain. The Dalai Lama has been quoted summarizing Buddhism in two words: "Everything changes."

In 2020 most of the worldwide population was faced with this reality, that many things they had taken for granted were about to change. The crisis wasn't so much the pandemic of COVID-19; it was our response to the virus, which we call in Buddhism the second dart of suffering.

The consumption of alcohol went up almost 100 percent in many parts of the world. Where I live in Vancouver, Canada, the rate of opiate overdose deaths surpassed the rate of deaths from COVID-19.

Fake news added to this second dart of suffering by promoting antimask campaigns and spreading news that it was a plandemic or a spamdemic. Sadly, some people believed this news so much that they ignored all precautions, and it has been claimed that some of those people ended up sick or dead from the virus.

The reality is that things have changed and continue to change. By the end of 2020 many places in the world required that we wear masks in public at all times, or we must take a COVID test to enter other countries. We gathered in numbers on Zoom and lined up outside stores, air travel slowed down, and we were unable to hug and hold our friends. Most tragically, families have been decimated by death and loss of employment and their homes.

All of this is painful, and we create a crisis when we are unable to accept that all of this has happened. How do we come into relationship with such painful realities?

The Buddha was an awakened spiritual teacher to some, a shaman to others, and a great healer to many. It can be said he provided a medical model for sickness, trauma, and crisis, known as the Four Noble Truths. The first truth describes the problem, which is suffering, a symptom of the human condition.

The Buddha taught that there would be pain—or more specifically *dukkha,* meaning unsatisfactoriness—because this body will age, get sick, and die. Hence viruses are part of the human condition. We have had them before, and another virus will come to plague us again. And in 2020, when most of the world was faced with this teaching daily, fear became a disembodied being for many, causing a daily crisis. Yet we have forgotten that there are countries where women don't even know whether their newborn will survive or if they will survive childbirth. We have forgotten that there are people who live under the daily threat of war, starvation, and natural disasters. And for them, this is just a reality, not a crisis. And some of us complain that we cannot leave our homes.

The second of the Four Noble Truths offers the diagnosis: craving, wanting a better experience.

The Buddha also taught that there was a path that led to more suffering. Throughout the pandemic, social distancing was one of the measures to help curtail the virus. There are people who railed against this, multiplying the suffering for others. Social distancing is a luxury for many of us; there are people who live in crowded homes and cities, where it is impossible to conduct spatial solidarity. Some of us in the BIPOC (Black, Indigenous, and people of color) and queer communities have experienced social distancing all our lives and have not protested against it. It has just been our reality.

The third truth offers a prognosis, the end of suffering. Perhaps it is not the hope we want because we will still age, get sick, and die.

The Buddha taught that there is an end to our suffering. This is perhaps the hardest truth to accept because the end can take months, years, decades, centuries. In 2020, we witnessed the destruction of the mythos in Western nations as hundreds of statues glorifying colonialism, confederation, slavery, residential schools, and oppression were toppled in one fell swoop. This followed the public lynching of George Floyd, and the response to this was wrathful action. The uprisings were liberation for many BIPOC people, and a crisis brought upon by systemic and institutional racism. Many BIPOC people have been campaigning for years to have these offensive statues taken down, and our requests have been ignored. Clearly, we needed the thunderbolt *vajra* action to cut through the hundreds of years of hatred, greed, and delusion. In Mahāyāna Buddhism, we call upon wrathful deities when needed. They are mostly needed to help calm the mind and emancipate the mind from the hell, titan, hungry ghost, animal, and god realms of the wheel of life that keep us enslaved in the prison of the minds. The symbol of the vajra sword is to remind us of the energy that is needed to cut through the chains of ignorance. An end of suffering does not mean we will avoid death. Death will come to all of us, some tragically killed or murdered, and others from the decaying body or natural disasters and accidents. An end of suffering is learning to meet all of this with compassionate equanimity.

The fourth truth offers the treatment plan. The Eightfold Path helps us alleviate the crisis and free us from the trauma of the second dart.

The Buddha taught there was a path that led away from suffering. He prescribed meditation, ethics, and wisdom. This three-part path, when fully lived, becomes the Noble Eightfold Path: Right Vision, Right Intention, Right Speech, Right Action, Right Livelihood, Right Effort, Right Mindfulness, Right Concentration. First, we must have the vision of something possible. Where there is vision there is the possibility of transformation. Transformation can happen when we pay attention to our ethical life of speech, actions, and livelihood. This helps us to progress along the path with a clearer conscience when we can wholeheartedly begin to embody meditation with effort, mindfulness, and concentration. This in turn can plow the ground for wisdom, whereby our vision and intention will flourish.

So, this is the remedy for crisis. Remembering that the crisis is not what happens to us. What happens to us is the first dart of pain. The crisis is the second dart. We suffer when we crave for a different experience, when we have aversion toward our experience. This causes a spiritual, emotional, mental, and physical crisis. When we turn toward our pain with compassion, and take the Noble Eightfold Path medicine, it will help to abate the crisis, leaving us with the pain, which is just part of the human condition.

We have a body; it will age, become sick, and expire. The best way to live is with the attitude that all plans are provisional. That everything changes. Once upon a time, the tiny island of England, a colonizing country, ruled the world. Then another colonizing country, the United States, began to rule the world. And now their rule over the world is weakening. It is a reminder that things do change. Nothing is permanent. I remind myself of this after every inhale and exhale move as I move closer to my demise. It is through transcending the second dart of suffering—which can be expressed as hatred, craving, and delusion— that we can begin to walk the path of freedom. A path where somehow, we have to learn to be with the pain of the first dart, without trying to soothe it with the second dart. The only thing that can soothe the first dart of pain is having faith that this too shall pass.

I offer this practice when we become caught up in the second dart of suffering. We can use this practice when we sit to meditate and find ourselves assailed by the proliferation of thought. The practice is called RUST. The mind can get rusty, causing it to function from a place of reactivity. If we can remove the RUST, we have the potential to act from a place of wisdom and compassion.

R: Relax and recognize what is activating you right now. Pause and really see if you can catch what is whirling around your mind. Recognize that whatever is activating you is full of subjective perceptions and judgments.

U: Understand that you are caught up in a story. A very old story. A story full of judgments, perceptions, resentments. A story that changes every time you replay it in your mind. Ask yourself, "Why am I still holding onto the story? What is it doing for me?"

S: Sit with the sensations in the body. Stand with sensations. Stretch with sensations. Sway the body with sensations. Sing with sensations or even silently scream with sensations. See if you can feel any tension or restriction in your body. What does it feel like? Where are the sensations located in the body? Place a hand where you feel these sensations and give this part of your body some kindness. Just know that the body is remembering past traumas, past hurts, past wounds.

T: Trust that this too shall pass. Trust that these sensations are changing all the time. You won't always feel this pain or discomfort. If the story of what happened is still playing in your head, tell it to be quiet. Ask it to relax, so you can let go of all the rust that has accumulated in your life—so you can be at peace.

Of course when we are activated or triggered we will never remember all of RUST. This practice is not linear. If we are triggered you may just call on U, and understand you are caught in the story. Knowing this can help you step out of the story. Or you may call on T, trusting that this too shall pass, or perhaps telling the story to relax, so you can have some peace. Or you may call on R, and recognize you have been triggered by something and need to do some self-care. Or you may just call on S, and allow yourself to sit with sensations, or stand, sway, sing, or scream.

RUST is another practice; it has the same taste of all the Dharma teachings. RUST has the taste of freedom, the capacity to free you from the prison of your mind.

4

CULTIVATING A SENSE OF IDENTITY

Won Buddhist Practice in Immigrant and Second-Generation Identity Crises

Hojin (Hye Sung) Park, PhD

One question most immigrants find themselves asking after coming to the United States is, "Who am I now?" They have embarked on a journey for a better life, but when they first arrive in the United States they feel like strangers, lonely and unsure how to fit in.

That is how it was for me when I first arrived. I could not drive nor speak English fluently. I needed other people's help to get anywhere. Then one day someone told me, "If you can't speak English or drive, you are handicapped in the United States. You can't do anything by yourself."

Feeling of Groundlessness

It was a new experience standing alone in a foreign country without family and friends, not having fluent conversations, nor the freedom to move around by myself. I found myself very far from the comforts I was so used to, and instead I was in a strange, awkward, and uncertain position.

It became harder to explain "Who am I now?" I started to search for my self-identity, wondering whether I was even the same person I was not too long ago. It was a feeling of being groundless, and I felt this same groundlessness when I interviewed first-generation Won Buddhist Koreans who had immigrated to the United States.

This confusion is even greater among second-generation immigrants born in the United States. You grow up in a Korean culture at home, but once you leave the doorsteps, you become an American. On top of that, if you are a Won Buddhist, you feel like a stranger, even to other Korean immigrants, since the majority identify as Christian.

I realized that there is a need for better understanding of Buddhist spirituality coping strategies and practices, including mindfulness and other sources of resiliency, during times of struggle for the Korean immigrant population. My doctoral dissertation, "Won Buddhist Coping in America Among the 1st- and 2nd-Generation Korean Immigrant Population," provided relevant research. The qualitative study was designed to gain a greater depth of understanding of the coping skills that Won Buddhist members employed. The sample for this study was the Korean immigrant Won Buddhist community in the United States. I conducted sixty- to ninety-minute face-to-face interviews with twenty-three participants. This study did not include people under age eighteen.

All adolescents struggle with self-identity during the awkward transition between childhood and adulthood, but this stage is so much harder for Korean Americans who are born and raised in Won Buddhist families. In the process of trying to find self-identity, some become rebellious while others mature and become more understanding and tolerant people. No matter, when we lack identity, we desperately long to understand who we really are. Many young immigrants are vulnerable to mental health problems, such as identity diffusion or low self-esteem, given that their immigrant parents may not be capable of providing support they need, due to their unfamiliarity with their new society and their own struggles with the hardships of immigrant life.

For example, I interviewed a young man who grew up as a Korean American in a city with barely any Asian population. Perhaps because of the subtle racism that still exists against minorities, he says he always felt alone, even when surrounded by others:

> It was probably when I was in middle school. Throughout my adolescent years, I felt intense loneliness and anxiety in my relationship with others. It was then that I sought Won Buddhist teachings to understand myself

better. I took the initiative to study the teachings because I wanted to find my self-identity.

Though his voice was composed, I could sense the loneliness behind it. Typically, once we figure out where we belong, we start thinking about how we can serve our family or our society. We find our life's purpose in these pursuits and increase our self-esteem as we receive acceptance and recognition from those around us. Therefore, the longer we stay in a state of loneliness and uncertainty in a foreign environment, the greater our desire to grasp who we are and where we belong.

Another young man who was born and raised in the United States had been struggling with conflicting identities within himself. His arguments with his parents represented a constant internal struggle between his two cultural personas. While East Asian culture places family and community above individuals, Western culture places individual happiness above all else. For example, any time he had a self-centered desire, it would be shut down by his guilty conscience, which stems from his deep-seated cultural obligation toward others:

> Living as a Korean American feels like I have two separate personalities in me. One is a traditional Korean eldest son and the other one is a typical American. I didn't even know I felt this way until I went to a university. In some areas, my parents and I can never reach an agreement because of the cultural difference. We have heated arguments because of these differences, and as they become more frequent, I get confused about where I really belong. This confusion still impacts my life.

The Role of Won Buddhist Meditation

When talking about mental health in an immigrant community, one must consider the cultural background as well as the generational gap in immigrant families. Second-generation immigrants are born in the United States to immigrant parents, while the 1.5th generation are children who were born in a different country, but immigrated to the United States at a young age. In a family where the parents are also struggling to fit into the new society, parents are often unable to help due to lack of finances or the language barrier. Children who grow up in these families tend to have deeper identity issues.

When asked how they overcame the struggle between multiple identities, most of these Won Buddhist young adults answered that they turned to meditation. Even meditating for a short period of time can restore a confused and anxious heart. In Won Buddhism, meditation is a practice that leads to the achievement of freedom of mind by gaining the ability to awaken to one's own nature, which is originally free from discrimination or attachment. The benefit of meditation is the attainment of peace in one's heart that isn't shaken by circumstances. Through meditation, one can find comfort in knowing the identity of one's consciousness that existed in the past, exists in the moment, and will continue to exist in the future.

Awareness of changes in mind and body is called mindfulness, which makes us calm, clear-headed, and steadfast. At times, we can focus on taking a deep breath in, or examine our breath as it is slowly exhaled. In this way, we can observe the changes within our body, emotions, and thoughts as an objective outside observer. The more we are able to look at ourselves objectively, the more we will be able to treat changes in our surroundings with courage and wisdom. Mindful choice in actions of daily life is emphasized in Won Buddhism. In practice, this means that mindfulness is more than maintaining present moment awareness. It also includes right choice in action, which refers to the intention of choosing what is just and forsaking what is unjust, with clear awareness during daily activities.

From those people who were interviewed, it was clear that mindfulness can help look into the changes in one's emotions and thoughts in the process of understanding one's self. For example, one of the interviewees said,

> The world continues to change. I believe that every change in this world can help me understand myself. So, when something happens, you can observe your own response. I ask myself, how am I responding to this matter, and what do I think about it? You can ask yourself these questions as well. Then you can look at why you think or act that way. Practicing mindfulness helps me understand myself whenever something happens.

Many feel anxiety and fear because everything is always changing. However, if we look at change as a path to understanding ourselves and for internal growth, we will feel our fear dissipate as we become more open-minded. Changes can be painful, but they can also be an opportunity. If we have the ability to objectively look at our physical and internal response through mindfulness, we won't be swept away by the changes, but instead, be able to find our true self amid the chaos.

How are second-generation immigrants applying Buddhism in their lives? One interviewee said that Buddha's teaching about impermanence helped. Impermanence simply means that everything in the world is always changing. Knowing that current circumstances will also inevitably change allows us to gain the strength to accept where we are, and learn from it.

This perception of the current situation anchors a person amidst constant change. The interviewee also said that this perception taught them to overcome external circumstances, instead of being controlled by them. Even though this person still currently struggles with self-identity and isolation due to racial and cultural differences, there is hope expressed in the fact that this would eventually change.

> Something that helped me about Won Buddhist teaching is that there is no cure-all answer to any situation. Everything is still happening and changing. There is no black-and-white answer to any situation. I do not yet understand everything from the Scriptures of Won Buddhism. However, what's important is that I learned to value the process of getting to the answer rather than focusing on the end results. I have learned to listen to my mind more carefully, and to do my best to organize my thoughts, follow through on them, and understand them. Everything is ongoing.

As this young man came to value the process more than the results, he obtained an open-mindedness about himself, as well as the conflicts within his family. Even if there is no immediate solution to a conflict, he strives to understand the problem better because he considers the process more important.

> I believe mindfulness is about changing habitual thoughts or actions that are normally done without awareness. For example, sometimes your road rage comes out when you run into someone who's driving poorly. However, if you practice mindfulness you can stay calm, rather than responding to anger right away. Sometimes, you can have someone in your family who's rather impatient that you get into arguments with. You can also use mindfulness in that situation to respond to their anger with calmness to avoid fights.

People who live mindfully tend to receive every moment of their lives as an opportunity to learn and grow with an open mind. If we can have a less stressful reaction when we don't have the final answer right away, we can create a way to step away from the anxiety and guilt of not being able to find the solution.

Bringing our unconscious to the surface is an important part of understanding ourselves. If we are mindful of actions or emotions that normally come up unconsciously, we could even change our subconscious bad habits.

Sometimes, you will find that there are suppressed emotions or unresolved problems that are translated into subconscious actions. When these problems remain unresolved, you can develop a habit of acting out offensively or defensively, without even knowing why you react in such a way. However, as you become more self-aware, you learn to reflect on yourself at every moment without being controlled by subconscious reflexes. Mindfulness helps in this process by enabling you to find your anchor.

It is a blissful thing to find an anchor within you that won't be shaken regardless of the outside circumstances. This enables you to actively respond to all the challenges you inevitably face in life, such as life and death, sickness and health, and good and bad circumstances. It is necessary to be on a journey to find oneself in a world where everything is constantly changing. And having the strength within your heart to face this truth is a necessary step to finding oneself and protecting your anchor.

Finding Self-Identity

Most second-generation immigrants find their self-identity as they pass from adolescence into adulthood. However, they experience many worries and internal conflicts in the process. As they start to find the answer to who they are, they become freer to talk about themselves and gain the confidence to discuss their experiences or beliefs with others. Similarly, self-esteem also grows as one gains the ability to freely express oneself and find the firm anchor of the mind through such mind study.

Mindfulness practice is related to finding our self-identity. As we continue to learn how to focus on the present and objectively observe changes in our emotions in various circumstances, we find out who we are, just as we are.

This perspective and understanding of self are unchanging despite external circumstances.

In this study, the term *mindfulness* is applied in four aspects: introspection, awareness, threefold study (virtue, meditation, and wisdom), and nurturing our Buddha Nature. Among these, threefold study and nurturing our Buddha Nature are also at the essence of Mahāyāna Buddhism—namely to cultivate wisdom and compassion. The aspect of "introspection" is about the careful observation of, and reflection on, one's own mind, emotions, and thoughts. This process is helpful for emotional healing and mental clarity. In Won Buddhism, mindfulness includes not only individual awareness, but also awareness of the larger conditions and surroundings, so one can think mindfully before putting thoughts into actions.

This young man also developed a deeper appreciation of meditation. "Through meditation and mindfulness, I do not let the external circumstances rule over me. They may be problems for me to work through, but not something that I should get swept up by. I believe this is how meditation and mindfulness empower you."

If we act on our emotions when we feel overwhelmed or uneasy, chances are that we will end up regretting our thoughtless actions. If we grow to observe our internal changes through meditation, we will find ourselves acting less by sheer reflex and instead learn to respond to situations more mindfully. On top of that, we will see our perspectives change during tough times and will learn to see that difficult external circumstances are not meant to put us in pain, but only to teach us to understand ourselves better.

Another person, who has been working in the United States and studying Won Buddhism for more than forty years, said that what changed the most is that, for him, Won Buddhism has evolved from something that he turned to only when in need to something that is a part of his daily life. In a similar way, a woman who immigrated to the United States over twenty years ago says there has been a change in her life as she pursued Won Buddhism in America. Before, she considered her religious life separate from her practical life. She focused on showing the good side of herself to others, but never regarded that as her true self. However, she says that over the years, despite her imperfections, her understanding of herself and love for herself grew, and that she is now able to accept herself as she is.

It takes time and effort for our religion and spirituality to become a part of our identity. One thing that deters this is when religion feels like a responsibility or duty rather than a source of genuine joy. Genuine joy or internal peace comes from how much we understand ourselves and others. Rather than ideological dogma, mindfulness focuses on the practical: on living out what we learn and finding out who we truly are—through self-awareness.

There are many reasons as to why crises occur and conflicts occur. But being bound to "What you should put your faith in" rather than "What kind of person you become through your faith" tends to worsen the conflict. What's truly important is how our religion increases self-awareness and helps people to live in awareness of self and others.

In addition to mindfulness practice, faith in the Dharma was equally as important as a coping skill for those Won Buddhists interviewed for this study. Many participants found peace of mind or comfort from their faith in Dharma and felt a sense of identity from their faith.

Empathy is the key to unity. There are countless examples of how empathy and understanding have turned a crisis into an opportunity for major growth. One such crisis is the acculturation process itself. Immigration is stressful for those who come from different cultural norms, languages, and social environments, and are now thrust into a new country. However, it could also become an opportunity for internal growth.

We can open the door to healing and growth when we use our understanding of our own pain and suffering to empathize with others. The journey to self-identity also starts here.

5

PSYCHOSPIRITUAL RELIEF WORK IN THE TSUNAMI AREAS AND THE POTENTIAL OF RINSHO BUDDHISM

Reverend Hitoshi Jin

On March 11, 2011, one of history's strongest recorded earthquakes struck off the coast of Miyagi Prefecture in northeastern Japan. This triggered an equally historic tsunami that devastated the coastal areas of three prefectures, reaching as high as a hundred feet, and traveling as far as three miles inland. On that day, about eighteen thousand people lost their lives with another five hundred thousand losing their homes. If this was not enough, these two natural disasters then caused the human-made disaster of the meltdown of three nuclear reactors at the Fukushima Number 1 nuclear complex, leading to a mass evacuation of the area and an ongoing legacy of suffering in the region.

To meet the tragic events of March 11, an outpouring of relief activities ensued by numerous Buddhist denominations, their youth associations, other smaller denominational groups, individual temples and individual priests, and Buddhist-based NGOs. Many Buddhist priests, not only in the disaster-hit areas but also in other parts of the country, held regular memorial services for those who perished in the disaster. As honoring the dead and revisiting grief through Buddhist memorial rites are a cornerstone of Japanese spirituality, Buddhist priests played an important role in helping many people face the massive grief brought about by the disaster. In the hardest hit areas, Buddhist temples acted as short- and long-term shelters for those left homeless by the tsunami. In Ishinomaki City in Miyagi Prefecture, four out of sixty-eight shelters were Buddhist temples, including the Sōtō Zen temple Dōgen-in. By the end of April, it had taken in 134 people and still hosted about 80 people into the summer months, until they moved into newly built temporary housing units in early August. In Kesennuma City, also in Miyagi, six out of seventy-seven shelters were Buddhist temples. Details of such activities by Buddhists during this disaster have filled dozens of volumes in Japanese, but this chapter will focus on the engaged Buddhist efforts of the Rinbutsuken Institute for Engaged Buddhism under the Zenseikyo Foundation & Buddhist Council for Youth and Child Edification. Of particular focus in this chapter is the issue of trauma experienced in disasters, a bodhisattva mindset that can ground care for such victims, and the particular activities that Rinbutsuken and Zenseikyo coordinated in response to the 2011 disaster.

The Rinbutsuken Institute and Zenseikyo Foundation: From Hosting Sunday Schools to Training in Psychospiritual Care

The Zenseikyo Foundation was established in 1962 and has a membership of over sixty denominations from mostly the traditional Japanese Buddhist world. Its purpose has been "to nurture young people in the spirit of Buddhism," and in the early years, it supported temples' efforts to establish Sunday schools and children's associations to cultivate young leaders. As times changed, it shifted its work to meet more recent pressing youth issues, such as school dropouts, bullying, and harassment. This led to engagement in even more critical issues, like *hikikomori* (shut-ins or social reclusion) and suicide. Out of this increasingly critical social work that went beyond the typical confines of Sunday schools and low-conflict social work, I spearheaded the formation of the Rinbutsuken Institute in 2008 to deepen the understanding of how to apply Buddhism to higher conflict and more complicated social problems. The Triple Disaster of March 2011 then pushed the institute even further to train and develop other Buddhist practitioners to engage in such high-leverage trauma, which included disaster relief care.

Before Rinbutsuken was established, I had worked for years in psychospiritual counseling for troubled youth and suicide prevention for Zenseikyo. During the 2011 disaster, I had to learn to adapt those skills to helping those in the disaster-stricken areas struggling with trauma and grief. However, after making extended visits to the three centrally affected prefectures of Fukushima, Miyagi, and Iwate, I saw that there was far too much work for Zenseikyo and Rinbutsuken to handle. While watching scores of Buddhist priests eagerly volunteer to perform memorial services and take part in material aid efforts, I felt an untapped potential in them to offer the kind of psychospiritual care for those who have experienced mass death and grief that only true religious professionals can offer. It was at this point that the Rinsho Buddhism Chaplaincy Training Program was born.

Using Rinsho Buddhism to Move from Trauma Care to Spiritual Care

There are various needs for a fundamental wisdom in the trauma care of disaster victims. Trauma itself can be explained as "the psychological state of an interruption or breach of trust between one's own self and the world outside." In other words, there is the feeling of loss about the possibility of living a normal life, experienced as "something is wrong." Concretely, this manifests in the loss of self-confidence to do something by oneself and the sense of betrayal by the world around oneself. This loss of trust leads to anxiety, such as, "What is going to happen now?" and "Am I going to be OK?" as well as the arising of despair, such as, "It's totally impossible now," and "It's impossible that things will get better."

Especially in the case of trauma caused by a disaster, it is easy for the feeling to arise: "I have been totally abandoned here amidst this very dangerous world." With the loss of a loved one related to trauma, in addition to normal grief, there are the continuing experiences of "intrusive memory," flashbacks, nightmares, and other experiences caused by past trauma, which feels psychologically threatening in the present. Victims can also suffer from thoughts like, "Couldn't they have avoided death?" and "What has finally come of them?"

In terms of responding to trauma, firstly, there is the attempt to remedy the situation in which the experience that has caused the trauma is reexperienced. Concretely, there is remedying the occurrence of flashbacks and the critical self-examination and strong psychological pain that is connected with events triggering the recollection of the traumatic experience, such as dreams and invasive memory. Secondly, there is remedying the problem of denial and paralysis. Concretely, we must not deny the importance of the experience by running away from it and becoming mindless through entertaining oneself constantly; we must ultimately face the reality of that experience. Thirdly, there is the problem of hyperarousal. Concretely, this expresses itself in insomnia and the inability to concentrate as well as being short-tempered and easily shocked. In the case of children, it can be accompanied by oversleeping.

When conspicuous obstacles continue to cause a hindrance for more than a month and PTSD arises, there is the need for support from psychological professionals. The main causes in the shift to PTSD are: the inability to gain support from others close to one, a high level of daily life stress, and the depth of trauma. Alcoholism, depression, and suicide are not uncommon in these cases, which were well documented in the Great Hanshin Earthquake Disaster of 1995.

There can be a great gap between individuals in how they experience and deal with trauma. Based on different mental and physical constitutions, the caregiver should put aside evaluations, because there is the possibility of repeating the trauma in the person; for example, the caregiver should avoid phrases like, "It's so sad"; "There are others with worse experiences"; "Please also do your best for those who died." If the victim internalizes the experience and trauma as their own personal matter, they can become very isolated. Especially for those who have lost a loved one, they may feel, "It would have been better for me to die too"—which is something that was often heard after the tsunami. Rather, the caregiver must become intimate with the victim's feeling, and by repeating this process of intimate interaction, gradually find a treatment that fits the victim.

Boddhisattva Responses to Trauma

For Buddhist priests in Japan, the most common opportunity to connect with people, especially those traumatized by loss and death, is at funerals and memorial services. In the weeks and months after March 11, it was heartening to learn directly from many of the victims in the disaster areas of their positive feelings toward Buddhist priests and their activities at this time, evidenced in such comments as, "Just listening to the voice of the Buddhist priests chanting saved me."

Buddhist priests, however, need to take such opportunities to go deeper into an intimate interaction rooted in active listening. In terms of Buddhist practice, this is related to the four practices of the bodhisattva *(shishohō)* in relating to people. The fourth such practice *(dōji)* is especially important as it refers to working together by putting oneself on the same level as others and participating alongside them in activities. This can be further explained as trying to understand the position of others and listening deeply without getting caught in a particular view. The idea is to listen as Kannon (Guan-yin) Bodhisattva would. It is not common, however, for most Buddhist priests to receive training in such deep listening, and this can be a high hurdle to get over for those whose training and conditioning involve only giving advice rather than listening and asking skillful questions.

A third practice beyond traditional memorial rituals and active listening is to encourage self-respect. Victims may have to learn not to compare themselves to others, no matter the situation, and to value the preciousness of their own existence. This idea is based on the story of the Buddha, who is said to have announced shortly after his birth, "I alone am the honored one in the heavens and on earth."

A fourth practice is to encourage an awareness of the connection of oneself to all sentient life in the universe. It is important to support the victim to reaffirm life, which is born from the connection to all the myriad forms, and to reaffirm the connection between oneself and one's family, friends, acquaintances, and nature.

A fifth practice is to encourage rebuilding karmic connections to those who have died. One can become aware of a connection to those who have died within oneself. However, it takes great power to heal trauma and grief. This involves connecting to a new identity by learning to live every day and developing the great fundamental power to move on from the past.

A final important topic in this process from psychological trauma care to existential spiritual care is the issue of death itself. In the disaster areas, we were sometimes asked by those who lost loved ones: "What happens after death?"; "Where does the spirit go to?" The answer may differ depending on one's faith or religion. However, it is important to habitually consider the problem of the afterlife and the problem of death. Especially when unaware of another's religious tradition or when you know it is different from your own, it's usually skillful to return such questions compassionately with another question. "What do *you* think happens after death?"; "What do you hope happened to your loved one's spirit?" Responses may differ, but my hope is that religious professionals will not balk, hesitate, or push these questions aside. They represent the innermost concerns of some people and reflect part of opening up to the caregiver. If religious professionals do not hesitate to take on these issues, victims will not lose the trust of others and the world outside. Especially for those who have lost loved ones, I think it can be a principal step in establishing a new individual identity.

Zenseikyo and Rinbutsuken's Post-Disaster Activities: Short-Term Relief Care

After the catastrophic events of March 11, Zenseikyo and Rinbutsuken quickly shifted their focus to providing various forms of support to the disaster region in northeastern Japan. We first conducted a three-week investigation and needs assessment in the region, and then we began providing material aid support among our member temples in some of the hardest hit cities, like Kesennuma and Ishinomaki in Miyagi Prefecture. We also mobilized volunteer priests from our network temples around the country and created caravans to deliver emergency supplies and cook hot meals.

In order to better develop our staff and volunteers for therapeutic work, we held four workshops from April to May on the topic "Introduction to Trauma Care during Times of Disaster" in Tokyo, Saitama, and Kyoto. Our workshop included a four-hour program consisting of a lecture on disaster trauma care, orientation to deep-listening volunteer work, a workshop on attitudinal healing, and a presentation on how to perform memorial services for the deceased. Among the 170 persons who attended these workshops, we were able to enlist 50 as staff to provide psychospiritual and religious care. They were dispatched at the beginning of May through July for two to three days every other week, visiting four or five shelters at a time. This first phase sought to deal with the initial trauma after the disaster and the adjustment to new lives in the shelters.

Zenseikyo first placed special emphasis for its trauma care on children in the disaster areas. There were children and youngsters living in emergency shelters who had lost family members and had seen shocking sights of death and carnage. They were suffering from insomnia and engaging in acts of violence toward others as expressions of their trauma. We first supported them by offering physical outlets through places to play. Many volunteers spent time with them doing play therapy through balloon art and providing punching bags on which to take out pent-up frustrations. While providing them with a means to play, we also sought to ascertain which children had active trauma problems.

The accumulated problems of living in the shelters—such as limited space to play and adults around them also experiencing increasing levels of stress with trying to rebuild their lives and locate missing relatives—often led to children developing secondary trauma or post–traumatic stress disorder (PTSD). The adults also fell victim to this secondary trauma, which was exacerbated by the particular culture of northern Japanese people, who have lived for centuries in small, isolated, and intimate communities. As such, they are hesitant to openly express their feelings and needs, especially to outside caregivers and helpers. Thus, from the beginning of May 2011, we entered another field of work to support adults through various forms of entertainment, such as movies, vocal concerts, performances, and so on. In this way, the initial emphasis was on supporting people through camaraderie and natural conversation rather than direct intervention or inquiry into their trauma. When formal activities are held, they are in the form of peer counseling in groups of people with the group leader acting as an active listener rather than a psychological counselor. However, much of the work is done in a more informal style through tea party *(ocha-kai)* events where people share time and conversation over tea and snacks.

Another special activity that we were involved in was mobilizing traditional forms of healing through the Japan Association of Biwa Onkyu Treatment Providers. They are a group based in Kumamoto Prefecture in southern Japan that specializes in a special form of moxibustion called *onkyu,* based on ancient Buddhist ayurvedic methods. Onkyu involves the heating of acupressure points and meridians through medicinal herbs, in this case the leaves of the Japanese *biwa* tree, which release the healing properties of the herb into the bloodstream. This work was especially amenable to the elderly, who make up much of the disaster area population. Being sequestered in shelters for long periods of time exacerbated the health problems of the elderly, who were not able to get enough regular exercise and also suffer from stress that induces high blood pressure, heart attack, and stroke. The treatment served as both a substitute care for people who had not been able to get their regular medicines and also as preventative medical and psychological care. This *onkyu* therapy helped alleviate both their physical and psychological stress.

Intermediate and Long-Term Relief Care

By September, all the emergency shelters were being closed, and those who could still not return home or find other housing were moved into temporary housing units. The temporary housing units can hardly be called houses. They were tiny rooms with no space to accept visitors. The compounds of such units of fifty or more contained one common building for meetings but very little space for people to use freely. As the cool weather and winter returned, the problem of the isolation of these remaining victims became a concern. Dealing with longer-term mental health issues during the long cold winter months in northern Japan became a serious concern. Compared to the surface-level immediate interventions mentioned earlier, this type of counseling required more intensive one-on-one work dealing with PTSD, depression, and suicidal tendencies. These concerns brought to the fore the need to refocus relief efforts on long-term mental health care for victims, care for exhausted relief workers themselves, and stronger coordination of all these services.

According to an investigation by Japan's public television network, NHK, by the end of September, ten people within the temporary compounds had died from the effects of isolation or from suicide. After their initial relief to survive the disaster, many victims faced the despair of trying to rebuild their livelihoods and their communities. From 1998 through 2011, Japan had a suicide rate of over 30,000 per year. Numerous government and NGO campaigns were launched to face this problem, including a network of Buddhist priests around the country. While the rate had dropped to 21,007 by 2021, this does not reflect increasing levels of mental health in Japan. Rather, it reflects the building of proper social safety nets to address it.

Beyond suicide and other mental health concerns for disaster victims, many relief workers were in need of their own care. Relief workers were stressed after months of continuous effort. They included caregivers working in refugee shelters, temple families who offered their temples as shelters, doctors and medical workers, and especially Self-Defense Forces soldiers who had to recover so many corpses from the coast after tsunami waters receded. They suffered from exhaustion, burnout, and trauma in their work.

As indicated, Zenseikyo and Rinbutsuken tried to help address these issues in numerous ways. However, even if there was a large cadre of Buddhist chaplains, the biggest problem in alleviating suffering within the disaster zone was the coordination of needs and services. Especially in the first year after the disaster, there was a dearth of people coordinating volunteers and matching skilled people to the areas where their skills and background were most appropriate. Many different individuals started projects to help, and denominations ran their own volunteer groups, but these efforts were not organized or synchronized. In this way, I focused part of my efforts on coordination. As Zenseikyo is a national organization supported by a wide variety of Buddhist denominations, I set up a dispatch center for Buddhist psychospiritual counselors in November to better coordinate such work in Sendai, the capital of Miyagi Prefecture and largest city in the disaster zone.

There was also a need for counselors and care providers to commit to the region. Because of the aforementioned barriers to outsiders coming in to help these local communities and the basic intimacy needed to do such counseling work, counselors could not simply come from other regions of Japan for two or three days at a time and expect to provide the needed level of care. Therefore, a more effective means was to train local Buddhist priests and family members in such counseling skills. Such local priests and temples have long-established ties to their communities and could most readily offer the kind of psychospiritual support people needed in the coming years.

There are only a limited number of individuals, however, who can go through more intensive professional counseling training, and the needs went beyond one-on-one therapy. Thus, Zenseikyo and Rinbutsuken were involved with a variety of other community-based activities. We held a short summer camp in August in Fukushima for seventy children and ten parents from the areas affected by radioactive fallout. Many other groups held similar such summer camps, including the Buddhist NGO AYUS's summer camp in Yamanashi, next to Mount Fuji, in mid-August. Such camps offered an outlet for children and an opportunity to reconnect, socialize, and play in larger groups again.

To help alleviate isolation issues of the middle-aged and elderly, Zenseikyo began in September 2011 to run herb tea café events in the temporary housing units. Either in the common community room or outdoors, we provided a space for people to gather to strengthen relationships among themselves and also to talk to our volunteers about their concerns. These were modeled loosely on the Zen tea ceremonies that the Sōtō Zen Youth Association established during previous disasters in other parts of Japan for supporting those living in temporary housing. One form of those gatherings is described in more detail in chapter 6 about Café de Monk. At our tea parties, we used Western herb teas that have medicinal and calming properties to support the well-being of those people.

Zenseikyo continues its work today through many initiatives that not only aim to care for those in crisis situations but also help train others to provide such care. Through Zenseikyo and Rinbutsuken, we created the Rinsho Buddhism Chaplaincy Training program that provides a mix of academic study and practical training. The program also emphasizes Socially Engaged Buddhist components by highlighting and examining the social systems and cultural values that act as sources of suffering and trauma in Japan. It exposes students to a wide variety of social issues that affect people, such as end-of-life care, suicide, youth problems like bullying, shut-ins (hikikomori), criminal behavior and reform, cults, poverty, community decline, disaster-related trauma, and even more politicized issues like nuclear energy. In the portions of training, there is more emphasis on developing deep listening skills and the reorientation of the religious professional from one who provides answers to one who supports victims to discover their own solutions through compassionate presence. While in recent years, the Interfaith Chaplain program has sought new venues for training their candidates beyond the disaster areas of March 11, 2011, the Rinbutsuken program was able from the start to access Zenseikyo and the Japan Network of Engaged Buddhism's vast national network to help candidates locate a variety of venues of training. We hope that those trained in both the above-mentioned ideals of bodhisattva work and the practical means to enact these ideals to serve those in various crisis situations will help create positive ripples that continue to impact this world for years to come.

This chapter was edited and prepared from two previously published articles: "The Potential of Rinsho Buddhism and Developing Buddhist Chaplaincy in Post 3/11 Japan" by Reverend Hitoshi Jin, November 28, 2012, and "Psycho-spiritual Relief Work in the Tsunami Areas: An Interview with Reverend Jin Hitoshi" by Jonathan S. Watts, November 2011, which was published in This Precious Life: Buddhist Tsunami Relief and Anti-Nuclear Activism in Post 3/11 Japan, *edited by Jonathan S. Watts (Yokohama, Japan: International Buddhist Exchange Center, 2012).*

6

CAFÉ DE MONK

Kaneta Taiō and the
Mobile Deep-Listening Café

Nathan Jishin Michon

One step into a back room of Kaneta Taiō's temple reveals he is not your average Zen priest. Various guitars and other instruments line the walls, along with plenty of recording equipment. He will often incorporate music creatively in the services he provides to surrounding communities. Whether teaching the Dharma, counseling disaster survivors, or leading those survivors through community activities, his creativity and humor perform a playful tango around his heartfelt sincerity and deep presence with others.

In many ways, the name of the movement he began reflects those traits: Café de Monk. The Japanese end nearly every syllable with a vowel sound, so the final word sounds more like "monku" than "monk." In Japanese, *monku* means "to complain." But in English, of course, *monk* can refer to an ordained priest. The Café de Monk reflects this play on words as "a place where those who need space to let off a little steam from their life can come and 'complain' to the volunteer 'monks' on hand." Kaneta also loves the jazz musician Thelonious Monk and incorporated him into the triple entendre of the café's name. He claims the loose and playful spirit of jazz guided their sense of the gatherings. Thelonious Monk's own "complex, here-and-there style fit the different emotions of people recovering from the trauma of a major disaster."

He had no particular training in deep listening skills or counseling when 2011's Great East Japan Disaster struck his home prefecture of Miyagi. His temple is in Kurihara City and survived with relatively little damage. But Kurihara is only about thirty to forty miles inland from towns like Ishinomaki and Minami-Sanriku, some of the areas hardest hit by the tsunami. In the immediate moments after the earthquake, all electricity in the region was out. Without any gasoline there, he could not leave that evening, and he was left to ruminate in the darkness about how the people in the surrounding areas were doing. He reflects, however, that in the following days,

> I began to hear about corpses from the coast being transported to the funeral home near my temple because the crematoriums and funeral homes on the coast were destroyed. I thought, "So many bodies are coming. This is probably more than the Buddhist priests close to the coast can handle. I have to at least be with these bodies as they're cremated and help with the memorial services." Thus, I began spending time with the grieving families. The first two deceased individuals who came in were both fifth-grade girls who I heard were good friends. My voice trembled as I tried to chant sutras for their funeral. I then continued to volunteer at the crematorium for the next two months, overseeing memorials for around three hundred people. During that time, roads to the coast began to be gradually repaired, and I was able to see and comprehend the extent of the destruction myself.[1]

As in many traditionally Buddhist countries, in Japan the forty-ninth day after death is considered important for a spirit moving on. Kaneta joined a large interfaith memorial service on the forty-ninth day after the disaster that included a Christian minister and priests from numerous different Buddhist traditions. They walked in a procession to the top of a hill overlooking the scene of destruction and chanted in a long line. The cherry blossoms had just begun to bloom during that time. He says that the sound of the chants turned into cries and yet, as that occurred, he could feel the lines between all their traditions fade away. "In coming face-to-face with the site of this tragedy, differences between our sects and religions had no meaning. I decided that the only important thing was to be with the suffering of the victims and face those truths together with them from whatever framework and understanding they stood upon."[2]

That experience helped inspire Café de Monk. This traveling café began with a small truck of supplies that ventured to different areas in the disaster-struck region. At first, however, there was not much deep listening, and the people who came did little talking. The disaster victims they met were not ready or willing to open up about anything. Especially in Japan, it is culturally uncommon to open up about your stress, anxieties, or traumas. As Kaneta explains, "We don't want to trouble the people around us by complaining about our own lives. So there is a tendency to hold that inside—especially around people you don't know very well."

At first, volunteer monks said things like, "We are ready to listen to you," "We'll provide mental care," "Go ahead and speak about whatever you like," but people said nothing in response. Thus, they began instead simply saying, "If you have the time, come be with us in a relaxed atmosphere." He made sure that volunteers never preached, spoke about sutra verses, or asserted the benefits of Buddhist practice. "We just tried to provide a comfortable setting where people could breathe and be in what way they felt they needed to, while we were available for support if desired." A café-type setting with drinks and snacks allowed an informal way for survivors to start a conversation with volunteers who are on hand to listen and be with them. Then, those who feel the need to go deeper into their experience can do so at their own pace and to a level that they are comfortable with. Kaneta learned through experience to become a better listener and helped volunteers to do so as well.

In order to create a space for listening, they first had to create a space that allowed for relaxing and loosening up. Thanks to the nonintrusive atmosphere, people gradually began to open up. Survivors who attended began to say things like, "Umm . . . Reverend, would you mind talking to me for a moment about . . ." Though Kaneta is quick to point out listening to these stories could be extremely challenging.

> At times, especially when starting out, I was stunned into silence. When an elderly woman talks about seeing their grandchild swept away, what can you say? There were some angry reactions. Numerous people asked me, "Who decided who lives and dies?!" There is no easy response for these expressions. I still waver, but would say something like, "You and I are both living, and there is definitely meaning in that. Let's work together to find that meaning."[3]

Kaneta paid more and more attention to people's subtle expressions, little murmurs, and slight facial movements. People sometimes say a lot without speaking. There is also plenty hiding behind the words they say. As Kaneta points out,

> Even when a person says "pain," ten different people probably use that word with ten different meanings. There is a story behind each of those words. To help truly understand what they are saying and to show them we are present, we have to listen not only with our ears but with our entire bodies.

He points out that Japanese has two different characters to write *listen* even though they are pronounced the same way. The first simply refers to the common idea of listening through the ears. But the second

> means listening with all your heart and mind throughout the body. The sound that enters our ears carries not only information, but emotion, the way of speaking, the intonation, and subtle senses that surround it all. We have to observe those clues carefully to truly listen. It involves listening with all our senses and our entire bodies. Without this, we can't get to the heart of what they are trying to convey.[4]

Café de Monk, however, is not always a somber place. Quite to the contrary, it is peppered with humor. Kaneta believes that humor is important in times of sadness and suffering. The play on words in the very name of the café tried to lighten the mood from the get-go.

> I like to play with words. One of the ways to refer to Buddhist priests in Japan, *bozu,* has the same pronunciation in Japanese as the popular music speaker company, Bose . . . Making little jokes while playing with words in the conversations helped to lighten the mood and loosen people's tension. Of course, you also have to be careful with humor. If you are perceived as making light of another's suffering, you can make their wounds cut even deeper than they already are. We have to also be careful not to assume that a joke that works in one situation will work equally well in another. But by reading the room and the atmosphere, it can be a great tool to loosen the tension in the air. Victor Frankl once said, "Humor is another of the soul's weapons in the fight for self-preservation." A good joke can actually connect to and sympathize with a person's pain. I think that humor done with deep listening is born in and for the present moment as an art of improvised love.[5]

Humor was only one tool to help make a space for people to relax and settle down. Volunteers served complimentary cakes and snacks, coffee and tea. They sometimes gave away donated flowers and art to brighten people's new shelter abodes. They played music, sang karaoke, and performed traditional group dances. There was a masseuse. They baked potatoes together.

Other activities were related to traditional spiritual beliefs. In Japan, the bodhisattva Jizo (Kşitigarbha) is thought to protect loved ones in the afterlife, especially children. So during some of the early Café de Monk setups, they helped people make their own miniature Jizo statues to honor the loved ones they lost. Volunteers also regularly helped people make their own prayer bead bracelets *(juzu)*.

Everyone ate and drank at tables together. Because all attendees experienced the same disaster, there was some sense of camaraderie and community while joining with others during the gatherings. This was important to prevent the sense of isolation that many felt after losing their homes and neighborhoods. Especially as time went on, the danger of depression and suicide continually increased as some individuals and families had to live for years in temporary shelters. "So we hoped," Kaneta says, "that these temporary café spaces could help bring some new sense of community to those in need of personal connection."

Although Café de Monk began as just several people and a truck traveling around a disaster zone, the need helped it continue to grow. They held regular meetings in community centers at shelters for the displaced people. When other disasters occurred in Japan, people began setting up a Café de Monk there as well. Now there are even a few permanent establishments that bear the name within elderly homes and hospices. No matter the setting, the drinks, snacks, and atmosphere help people to settle down enough to express what's inside, and when they are ready, volunteers are available to listen with their entire being to the issues at hand.

7

LOTUS IN A SEA OF FIRE

The Hong Kong Case in 2019 and 2020

Chun Fai (Jeffrey) Ng

While the whole world faced waves of social movements and pandemic outbreaks during 2020, Hong Kong has been on the frontier of the battles for democracy and health since 2019. The Anti-extradition protests began in June 2019 and provoked plenteous international reactions. Then, the territory was among the first few places in the world that reported the first batch of confirmed cases of COVID-19 in late January 2020. Meanwhile, one out of seven Hong Kong citizens identifies themselves as a Buddhist. As the Sixth Patriarch of the Chan School of Buddhism says in the Platform Sutra, "Dharma can only be found in the world, and enlightenment cannot be attained away from it." There are real-life teachings in Hong Kong on how Buddhism can be the raft through the storms of crises.

I will start by depicting a general picture of mental health in Hong Kong over the recent crises. I will then analyze how psychological suffering comes about from the point of view of the Saṃdhinirmocana Sutra. Lastly, I will propose that the solution to the crises in society is the way within—how we can mend separateness in society through a correct understanding of the doctrine of dependent origination and reconstruct values through implementation of the bodhisattva ideal, so that each of us has the potential to transform ourselves and rebuild society into a Pure Land.

General Observation: The Psychological Suffering of the People of Hong Kong

The Department of Psychiatry at the Li Ka-shing School of Medicine of the University of Hong Kong conducted a survey from February to July 2020 involving 11,493 participants who are members of the general public in Hong Kong. They reported that 41 percent had moderate to high levels of post–traumatic stress symptoms and 74 percent had moderate to high levels of depression, no matter whether the participants supported or opposed the social movement. These mental health issues can be largely attributable to two major factors: breakdown of social connections and collapse of common values.

Social relationships are falling apart throughout the Hong Kong social movements, worsened by the occurrence of the pandemic. The protest has been overshadowed by a form of identity politics that dehumanizes a person into a mere label of their political stance: the "yellow-ribbon" camp stands for pro-democratic movements, and the "blue-ribbon" camp consists of pro-establishment supporters, the counterprotesters. Such division and polarization among people with different political views, fueled by a mere label, have caused alienation and conflicts in social groups and disintegrated friendships, families (parents are usually "blue-ribbon" while their children are usually "yellow"), working relationships, and even large sectors of society—the Yellow Economic Circle grew as a collection of businesses openly promoting protest messages. There is a prevailing distrust among citizens toward each other, the government, and the police, and there seems to be no buffer zone between the two extremes. With the outbreaks of COVID-19, face-to-face interactions have been largely reduced, and social distancing measures have aggravated the issues of isolation and exclusion.

Without social trust and sufficient social resources, emotional issues escalate. Throughout the protests, myriad heartbreaking and saddening events happened, like sieges of the universities and police crackdowns, which have drastically changed the lifestyles of the citizens and shaken the fundamental and traditional value systems of both camps. The blue-ribbon camp believes protests have made social stability and financial prosperity fade away, while the yellow-ribbon camp thinks the suppression of the protests and the subsequent implementation of the national security law subvert justice, liberty, and democracy. Many Hong Kong youths mourn the "dying of the city" and suc-cumbed to despair, hopelessness, and powerlessness. Such witnessing and expo-sure to the occurrence of those traumatic events in person or through the spread of information over social media, and the consequential subjective perception of the collapse of value systems, have produced various forms of emotional dis-tress, such as depression, anxiety, and even collective trauma. Worries around the pandemic outbreak again have exacerbated mental health issues.

Suffering Comes from Imprecise Understanding of the Nature of Things

The Buddha said repeatedly through the sutras that what he teaches is about suffering and the cessation of suffering. The core teachings of the variants of Buddhism today are inseparable from their ultimate concerns: human suffering and its cessation. They differ only in their perspectives, focuses, and levels of profoundness. Regardless of the external circumstances, which only act as the trigger, many Buddhist teachings assert that our own suffering stems from our flawed view of the nature of phenomena and ignorance of what reality truly is.

The Saṃdhinirmocana Sutra, one of the primary texts of the Yogācāra tra-dition of Mahāyāna Buddhism, provides us with a perspective on the nature of phenomena. In the sutra, the Buddha presents to the bodhisattva Gunakara the threefold nature of phenomena as the Three Natures: the Fabricated or Imagi-nary Nature, the Dependent Nature, and the Perfected Nature. It is said that if we can truly discern these three ways of understanding the nature of phenom-ena, we can reflect and deepen our understanding of all situations in life and thus liberate ourselves from suffering.

Imaginary Nature refers to us imposing names, labels, symbols, or ideas to the essences, attributes, and inherent being of phenomena so as to subsequently designate a convention. Such imputation is useful for our communications in daily life because it is almost impossible for us to complete a task with others without the use of words, language, descriptions, and concepts. The problem is that we cling to such conventional designations that we have imposed as the essences and attributes of the phenomena, which are illusory. If we cling to con-cepts, we tend to think of things in a certain reifying way and apply essences to phenomena to make things appear to be independent and separate.

One of the important functions of a symbol in a social campaign is identification, which allows cohesion among the movement's participants and creates distinction between insiders and outsiders. Another function of symbols is sanction: the institutionalized use of the symbol in promotional materials and displays, which gains group members' support and approval for the organization. Such conceptual grasping provides our minds with a very convenient but oversimplified way to process information and identify whether another individual is an ally or a threat so that we can instantly decide, and at the same time enhance alienation between insiders and outsiders, with the ultimate aim of maintaining and protecting our self-identity and ensuring our survival.

On the flip side, we might overemphasize the value of such names and symbols, which are mental constructs that don't have real substance or independent reality. This is what has led us to fall victim to manipulation and to reduce the wholeness and humanness of a person into a mere label, and to believe that the label is real and the person is an entity entirely separate from myself.

The labels themselves are not the problem. Our attachment to the labels and attributing essences to the labels are. Yellow ribboners believe they fight for freedom and democracy, the core values of Hong Kong, and to maintain their identity as a Hong Konger. Blue ribboners believe they protect the prosperity and stability of Hong Kong and maintain the current lifestyle. Our identity as a Hong Konger is also a mental construct that is subject to our individual identities, developed with different demographics (educational background, income, social class, and age). It is almost impossible for us to define what a Hong Konger truly is unless we put ourselves in a box and become attached to it. Such attachment to mental labels leads to imaginary separation between "me and allies" and "you and enemies," and it manifests as divisiveness in society. Hatred in the community is a natural result because each of us is fearful, even if unconsciously, of the erasure of our identity, both individually and collectively. We are then inclined to protect and sustain those identities through, among other ways, defeating the out-groups.

The solution can be put simply as "see labels as labels." We mistakenly narrow our scope of awareness and reduce another person to the mental labels in our mind. When we reidentify that each of us is of the same nature, it is far easier to wish another person to be physically and mentally well with joy and peace. Helping and offering assistance can become nearly automatic. Enlightened persons see projection as characterless, so that they do not confuse mental constructs with reality and are not caught in the afflicted character. It is only by recognizing that the labels, "yellow" or "blue" or the value systems that they symbolize, are of no permanent essence that we can liberate ourselves from indulgence in the illusory constructs.

One exercise I found very useful is contemplating that another person is just like me—all sentient beings at some point in their life are going through frustration and joy, and they wish to be happy and free from suffering. Regardless of how different our appearances, personalities, and political stances are, that person has the same nature as me, regardless of appearances and expressions. This breaks down the illusory barrier between me and that person (and other sentient beings).

Healing Separateness in Society: Understanding Dependent Origination

If we are able to understand how our suffering comes from attachment to self-created mental constructs, what is the nature of things happening in our life? Just like all schools in Buddhism, the Saṃdhinirmocana Sutra explains how dependent origination is the arising and ceasing of every worldly phenomenon that depends on other causes and conditions. In the face of divisiveness in society, we tend to assume, erroneously, that every person or every individual political group can be cut off from the other members of the community. The doctrine of dependent origination tells us that is impossible because our survival relies on the infinite, untraceable, and collective actions of others. Separateness is not the way; it is about co-creation. In the face of powerlessness, we have mistakenly ignored that we are not on our own but rather are inextricably connected to others.

When I realized that, I felt comforted, but still tried my best to do things that needed to be done *without being attached to the result*. When I came to terms with the fact that I have no control over the results of an external event, paradoxically, I felt *more* empowered and energized. Surrendering control is not a weakness but a strength: it means the extinction of separate selfhood and relinquishing the ability to plan and control external events.

There are three implications of the doctrine of dependent origination:

1. Everything is an ungraspable, inconceivable, and inexhaustible mystery that does not arise from a single cause or condition.

2. Everything is inseparable from everything else and is therefore interconnected.

3. Everything is subject to impermanence and is beyond absolute control.

In the following paragraphs, I will describe how contemplation of these three implications of the doctrine can transcend certain unpleasant emotions. Also, based on the doctrine, each of us represents an individual dot, yet we are interconnected with each other in the infinite net of human civilization. By transforming our own psychological suffering and transcending perceived separateness, we react with each other and transform society as a whole.

First, everything is a mystery in the sense that without using language and superimposing concepts, we cannot describe and understand what a phenomenon truly is. In other words, a phenomenon can only be understood by direct contemplation. Therefore, it is impossible for us to attribute the start of the social movement or the detriment of society to one single cause, like the government, the protesters, or the police. However, we are often subject to single-cause fallacy—we attribute blame to a single or limited number of causes. When we can attribute the cause of a mishap to a culprit, we perceive that we can simplify the complexity of an event and rationalize it to alleviate anxiety about our cognitive inability to comprehend the innumerable causes for the occurrence. The result is that, in contrast with our expectations, external blame leads to an increased level of anger, guilt, and hopelessness, and that is predictive of depression.

In the beginning, I always felt angry about the unfairness and unreasonableness of things happening in Hong Kong. In contemplating the Dependent Nature, I realized such anger came from the differences between the reality and my clinging to specific beliefs about how things should have worked in Hong Kong, and the unchanged value systems that we should defend. My attachment to such a misconceived story prevented me from looking objectively at what was actually happening. Such anger was derived from the fear of the collapse of my belief systems and the current lifestyle around me, and ultimately it stemmed from ignorance of reality. When I understood that things just happened, like a mystery but not specifically *to me* or to anybody else, and that it was only under my fixed mindset that things appeared to have moved against my illusory wishes, my anger subsided.

Second, by recognizing the interconnectedness among different people in society, we can both transcend our emotions and also help to heal the separateness. Our moment-to-moment existence is interdependent with numerous causes and conditions. Our life is powered by others. If someone believes in the self-sufficiency of the Yellow Economy Circle or selective enforcement and disproportionate use of force against protesters are the only solution to the social unrest, these ideas assume a false separation among people in Hong Kong, which will lead to distressing emotions and then unskillful behaviors. Acting out these emotions would unavoidably cause more suffering to ourselves, even though it seems we have the self-righteousness to do so.

When we realize our existence depends on the power of others, we let go of grasping for separateness and recognize that every person is inevitably interconnected with every other. By dissolving the division between self and other, we liberate our minds to realize that we have never existed as isolated islands. This reminds us of the true motivation of a social movement—for a better world, inclusive of all walks of life and all types of sentient beings, out of compassion. We can *then* approach the movement with wiser action and engagement.

Third, since dependent origination means that phenomena rely on other causes and conditions, there is nothing that can be produced and sustained by itself. When the causes and conditions change, the phenomenon will disappear. Even our existing lifestyles and value systems are unstable and cannot be relied on.

Guilt, hopelessness, and powerlessness were common emotions experienced by Hong Kong people during these two years. Guilt came from the belief system of "not doing enough to save the situation." Hopelessness came from the belief that "things will never be the same" or "unjust things will stay the same in the future." Powerlessness came from "uncertainty about what to do to change the situation." Under the doctrine of impermanence, everything is alive and in constant flux in every present moment, and everything is unpredictable and unreliable. On one hand, we have allowed our happiness to be dependent on external circumstances, and on the other hand, we have overestimated our power to control the event. The social movement is also dependent on the rise and cessation of numerous causes and conditions. One's actions, which are only one of the infinite conditions, are inseparable from the actions of others. The occurrence of an event actually depends on the actions of others. As I mentioned before, when I realized these factors, I felt comforted but still tried my best to do things that needed to be done *without being attached to the result*. When coming to terms with the fact that we have no control over the results of an external event, we can actually feel more free, more empowered, and more energized. Thus, surrendering control is not a weakness but a strength.

Value Reconstruction Based on a Bodhisattva Ideal

Often we are anxious about not being able to do something to change society. A more in-depth question is, From what value systems do our actions come? Following the collapse of prevailing value systems today, can some values in Buddhism be useful to humanity? Can we borrow them to reconstruct our existing value systems in a more sustainable and satisfying way?

The teaching on the Perfected Nature of reality describes the "suchness" of phenomena—things as they really are. One analogy to understand this is a mirage. Mere conceptual grasping is the belief that the mirage is real water. The Dependent Nature is the mirage itself. The Perfected Nature of reality is the emptiness of both the mirage and the observer. The water is viewed as just water without a mental construct and differentiation between the self and the perceived object.

Human beings constantly strive to understand the world around them, and this imposing of meaning onto the world is a goal in itself and a spur to action. In fact, every human action involves making meaning. What's special about a social movement is that it actively creates meaning and challenges meanings established by dominant norms and social institutions. A twenty-five-year-old Hong Kong activist was once interviewed by Reuters, and said, "My dream is to revive Hong Kong, to bring a revolution in our time. . . . This is the meaning of my life now."

Emptiness is not philosophical nothingness, but full of aliveness that gives rise to phenomena. As the Heart Sutra asserts, form is emptiness and emptiness is also form. If we are attached to the idea that life has no meaning, we fall into the trap of nihilism. Meaning is us imposing our ideas and values onto life, which can be purposeful and beneficial to the well-being of all sentient beings. Therefore, the issue is, What kind of meaning are we searching and striving for?

Korean Seon (Zen) Master Seung Sahn once said,

> Human life has no meaning, no reason, and no choice, but we have our prac-
> tice to help us understand our true self. Then, we can change no meaning to
> Great Meaning, which means Great Love. We can change no reason to Great
> Reason, which means Great Compassion. Finally, we can change no choice to
> Great Choice, which means Great Vow and the Bodhisattva Way.

The essence of Mahāyāna Buddhism can be described in two words—*wisdom* and *compassion*—and they are inseparable. Chan Buddhism considers wisdom and compassion to be inseparable wings of our true nature. Social justice and benevolence are ways to express compassion, but they should be accompanied by wisdom, the correct understanding of phenomena as emptiness, and transcending boundaries between the self and others. Simply put, wise compassion is a complete understanding of the true nature of common humanity. If we realize our own true nature, compassionate acts are a natural expression.

Sentient beings suffer because they are yet to realize the true nature of phenomena. A bodhisattva is a compassionate being who has embodied wisdom and vowed to save sentient beings from the sea of suffering because of deep love for them. The bodhisattva understands that all sentient beings are of the same nature as they are and has a profound awareness of their suffering.

The historical Buddha was indeed a compassionate social activist. He promoted the formation of the Sangha out of the caste system. He openly opposed ritual sacrifices. He also tried to dissuade rulers from waging war on neighboring kingdoms. Buddhism itself is a catalyst for social transformation against social injustice. I believe the original intention of most social movements is to improve the livelihood and well-being of people in the world. The difference in Buddhist values–driven social action is whether we have the "right view" toward these worldly events—whether we have a correct understanding of the nature of phenomena. If we do not have the right view of what is happening now, no matter how glorified our intention is and regardless of our political stance, our actions out of flawed views and their emotions will eventually lead us and others into more suffering. Thich Nhat Hanh said that hatred, violence, and anger can only be neutralized and healed by one antidote: compassion.

Compassion can be divided into different levels. Listening to another camp's opinions, with an open and nonjudgmental attitude and radical acceptance, while maintaining a clear understanding of our own and the other person's feelings and perspectives, is already an act of empathy and compassion. This does not mean glossing over differences—we can appreciate the differences in others while seeing the same fundamental humanity underneath.

A relation-oriented type of meditation, such as loving-kindness and compassion meditation in Theravāda and Tibetan traditions, emphasizes nurturing harmonious relationship with ourselves and others. Practicing this type of meditation leads to cognitive reappraisal and new perspectives, which means diminishing intergroup bias, generating positive emotions, and enhancing well-being through exploring meaning in life. Moreover, it also enhances social connectedness and lessens social isolation. These improvements are crucial in mending the enlarging social divisions in Hong Kong and other parts of the world.

The Way Within

There were some criticisms of Buddhist organizations in Hong Kong for their inaction when compared with other religions. Despite the large number of self-claimed believers, the Buddhist community in Hong Kong is scattered and perceived to be apathetic to political conflicts because of its spiritual emphasis and other pragmatic concerns. I reckon the more profound explanation is differences in worldview. The Avataṃsaka Sutra asserts, "If people indeed wish to know the Buddhas of the three time periods, they should contemplate the nature of the Dharma realm; all is but mind's creation." The historical Buddha is a unique psychotherapist, and Buddhist enlightenment is considered a radical and ultimate transformation of the mind. As Thich Nhat Hanh puts it, "The way out is in."

Societal transformation starts by understanding how the mind actually works and enhancing the quality of its functions, resulting in improving our thoughts, emotions, and behaviors. The origin of Humanistic Buddhism was a reform at the beginning of the twentieth century in China to reintegrate

Buddhist practices into everyday life and shift the focus back to the living, which has inspired many Han Buddhist organizations in Hong Kong today. Notwithstanding the escalating scale of charity and disaster-relief work performed by these organizations, the emphasis always comes back to practices to cultivate wholesome qualities of the mind, especially during times of turbulence.

Psychotherapy methods nowadays share an emphasis on the present moment and make use of secularized mindfulness practices as one of the interventions to purposefully direct clients' attention to the experiences of the present moment, without judgment, so that clients can cultivate a more receptive attitude to life's experiences. Mindfulness practices are particularly useful these days and are promoted widely by nongovernmental organizations as a tool of emotional management and regulation. However, there have been growing criticisms that mindfulness has become merely an objectified technique to enhance productivity in capitalistic society, with its moral and ethical essence in Buddhism stripped away, including a correct understanding of karma and the quality of wisdom and compassion. It is the cultivation of these values that brings transformation to us and to others in society. The techniques are only a vehicle. It is not necessary to expound these values in religious jargon, but they are crucial as fundamental values to humanity as a whole.

Some mindfulness practice groups in Hong Kong that focus on youth education have been pivoting from technique-oriented to value-oriented emphasis. In the beginning, these groups focused on integrating mindfulness techniques during participation in social initiatives. Then they figured out how psychological transformation and emotional care are more appropriate responses to alleviate the suffering from collective trauma, and they created enhanced practice sessions and workshops in deep listening and cultivating empathy and compassion. They have recognized that the practice of Buddhist ethical values in everyday life is already a radical social movement and transformation. Thich Nhat Hanh once asserted that without suffering there is no way for us to cultivate understanding and compassion. Being engaged in a social movement, even witnessing such a movement, can raise consciousness and result in transcendent learning, since we can critically examine assumptions, perspectives, and values that have influenced our approach in exploring the meaning of life. During the pandemic outbreaks, all practice sessions were conducted online. This was a silver lining in that reduced social interactions allowed youngsters space to calm down, restructure their daily routines, and make use of mindfulness practices as a means of self-discovery and understanding the world—both inner and outer.

The Chan School of Buddhism does not see practices as an instrumental intervention tool. It sees life as practice and practice as life. Contrary to the common understanding that Buddhist practice is the path to liberation, the Chan School considers enlightenment not an external attainment through practice but a practice itself. Everything is "suchness," which is always perfect and complete; practice is not only a means, nor simply a process to enlightenment, but both a means and an end in itself.

Pure Land Is Here and Now

The Vimalakīrti Nirdeśa Sutra says, "If a person's mind is pure, he will see the merit and magnificence of this land." Instead of only blaming the outside world for our own suffering, we can take responsibility of our well-being and change. Responsibility here means "response-ability." If we can understand and realize more about the true nature of ourselves and worldly phenomena, we may be able to take appropriate actions in response to whatever situations arise, which ultimately leads to transformation of our own self and society as a whole.

8

FINDING FLOW IN CRISIS

Dr. g

The Update

For hundreds of years, Black people across the diaspora have been stripped of their rooted names and given the surnames of slave owners, labeled as less than human, and priced with arbitrary labels to benefit the economy of white supremacy. We have been treated as currency, not the essence of the gods as we were designed. Black people spend considerable energy holding their definition of self because they are inundated by the definitions of others. In spite of this, somewhere between the inhale and the exhale, somewhere in between the end of the workday and crossing the threshold of one's home, Black people have found a way to continuously realign to the truth of their humanity, regardless of dominant spaces and ascribed definitions.

As the trail of pheromones that once wafted from sports, entertainment, and travel temporarily faded, many people across the globe were forced into their homes. For the first time for many this created a tighter silo to observe the degeneration and delight of the Earth, the mastication of society, one's family patterns and habits, and the wildness of one's mind. In the United States, where we will focus the attention of this discourse, people were in isolation or limited pods and inundated with the image of the dead Black body, like the days of lynching. Since the 2014 shooting of Michael Brown, an unarmed Black man from Ferguson, Missouri, to the 2020 murder of Breonna Taylor, in bed at her Louisville, Kentucky home, we have watched police person after police person acquitted. Between 2015 and 2020, there were 126 unarmed Black people killed.[1] Less distraction allowed the toxins of the nation, racism, and white supremacy to seep to the surface with no commercial break. Many people began to be exposed to the ways the system was killing innocent people and promoting inequities, how they benefited from it, and that it was part of their lineage. Racism was their system, and they had to come to terms with the ways they were upholding a system today that caused not only oppression but the innocent death of a representative of the global majority; of focus here, Black people.

> every fault is in fashion
> grab your gear
> t-shirts
> black lives matter
> are poppin' this year.
> pitch a sign for the yard
> or windowsill:
> we practice kindness; all are welcome; we do not kill
> every fault is a fashion
> and Guilt   is trending.

The Crisis

Crisis. *Noun.*

1. a time of great danger, difficulty, or doubt when problems must be solved or important decisions must be made

2. a time when a problem, a bad situation, or an illness is at its worst point[2]

The service I have offered over the last fifteen years has been inextricably tied to who I am on Turtle Island (the United States). As a first-generation female-bodied Caribbean Black, I was raised with a sense that our mind, the Caribbean mind, was different from the African American mind: we were free to create our own worlds by our own definitions. Yet, being nonbinary and queer was viewed as an abnormality. Regardless of my internalized racism, I experienced, missed, and witnessed many atrocities connected to racism, from profiling to loss. The mind and spirit were always my preoccupations, so I survived to complete my doctorate in clinical psychology and, after a ten-year dive into the practice of Buddhism, a chaplain. In that time I have worked within numerous facilities and my own space with hundreds of BIPOC (Black, Indigenous, and people of color), from troubled youth to the dying. Along this path, moving through crisis, being able to sense into its rising, and helping others through it was a charnel ground I slowly accepted as home.

Before 2020 I would have said few in the United States kept an ongoing awareness of the historical crises the global majority faced on a daily basis. From the treatment of immigrants and refugees to the detainment of Mexican children, the sense of urgency has often lulled to the background. The inhumane treatment of Black lives has been an alarming crisis point for hundreds of years. Therefore, I will focus this discourse on Black lives and experiences. Although this urgency has coursed through the blood and bones of generations of Blacks, concurrently the white majority has stayed ignorant to these truths and the key role they play in the intergenerational suffering of others. Only now are the white majority seeing their part in the impact of racism on another member of the human species. Still, the more the intersecting identities, the harder it seems to see the fullness of the Black human being before them.

your crisis. Our normalcy.

Every system is being challenged to dismantle harmful oppressive social structures and oppressive hierarchies to make way for the freedom of full being. The QTBIPOC and BIPOC at other intersections in my practice are challenging external systems that no longer serve them, internal systems that they have integrated as part of their self-identity, shadow systems that are felt and seemingly nameless.

We need all sides to change: the oppressor to free oppression as their weapon and the oppressed to accept change. Black people hold both sides within. Many Black beings have internalized unhealthy ways of surviving the system, such as the normalcy of mania, the us-versus-them, seeming glorification of the lack of self-care, inability to measure what is enough, focus on what we didn't do or accomplish, future-tripping, and in constant comparison by the measure of expectations set by the white majority. Black communities also continue to work with accepting intersections of our identity, particularly around gender identity, polyamory, or gender roles. If we are to get free, we also have to work on accepting all intersections of Black identity.

In essence, the lineage of the master continues and finds new language, even masked behind shouting for BLM (Black Lives Matter). In addition to navigating the dreams, the blood and sweat of cultivating a rich and equitable society, and balancing internal stresses, there is the added pressure of raising the awareness of others. This latter stress has left many of my clients being harvested for their experience, to grant emotional stability alongside the push to produce and "keep the economy running." Promotions and new job titles tasked Black people to eradicate a racism they did not create. And in the backdrop, the COVID-19 pandemic was impacting Black bodies at significant proportions. We cannot continue to burden a people already burdened by a broken system.

The Flow

The ground with my clients has been finding creative ways to be whole and to see their Being as more than how they are defined in society. This involves cultivating a mind that allows for expansiveness to see the ways our Being is inseparable from all that surrounds us, both what is rejected and what is missed. In order to achieve a sense of freedom, a freedom beyond any law or rule of humans, we must free the mind. It is the path of spiritual warriorship to deeply befriend this human experience, while also remembering that our essence expands far beyond the limits of our definitions or those imposed by others. We have been so focused on social liberation—on lasting change in social systems—that we bypass ultimate liberation, the freedom of mind that sees the innate abundance and connectedness of all things. We have the capacity to hold and fight for both.

The Three Doors of Liberation

Why is this Dharma, these teachings, for Black people and BIPOC? My clients are bodhisattva warriors. Bodhisattva warriors are those sentient beings who recognize their essence is enlightened and delay their own nirvana, their own liberation, to work to save all others who have not seen the truth of their Being. In essence, they hold the view that their liberation is inseparable and intricately connected with your liberation. As warriors, they are nonviolent and use weapons of generosity, patience, exertion, meditation, discipline, and wisdom to accomplish their activity. The fervor and drive of their activity are needed, but just as much, what is needed is their lives. We are slowly beginning to drift from the ways of our activist ancestors who ran themselves into the ground. In order to help others help the cause, one must see the self as the other and care for themselves, or find support to care for themselves. We cannot do it all, nor is doing it all a marker of success. As we move from the model of a centralized figure in charge of a movement, we can share the load in responsibility and rest. This is not a sprint, it is a marathon, a generational marathon. In order for it to last beyond the generations of oppressive institutions, we need to rest, reflect, and sharpen our mind, body-speech, and spirit toward liberation.

The first door of liberation is emptiness. No self. Often when we hear emptiness, we think that something does not exist. We absolutize and cling to our identity, denying the impermanence and ultimacy of this form. When we say no self, we are saying that our sense of "I" is not separate from things around us but inter-being (a term coined by Thich Nhat Hanh). The practice then is to loosen our fixation on the concept of a separate me that excludes others and inevitably leads to suffering. It is to ask the question: How am I connected to who or what surrounds me? Here we have an opportunity to see the ways our Being is interconnected with, say, Nature and its abundance, rather than the limits of racist terminology.

The second door of liberation is signlessness. The Buddha said to Subhuti, "In a place where there is something that can be distinguished by signs, in that place there is deception."[3] The Black identity has been normed with fixating on white frames as the ground of who they are and how they define themselves. It has been such that many hold tension because they have another way they would like to Be. Being comes at the risk of vulnerability, the risk of harm, the risk of resistance, to losses of material sources of well-being. It becomes easier to find the white frame and fashion oneself around it. Trim off the rest. The practice of signlessness is to open to new forms. To open to knowing and seeing the ways things don't die; rather, they transform. Our work is to see that the entirety of our Being is neither a snapshot of our experience nor the moment-to-moment changes in body, thought, or feelings.

The third door of liberation is aimlessness. When have we given ourselves permission to move through this life without a goal, without some sense of striving? This is living a life of future-tripping. Sometimes we call it the hustle. Here again is another other-defined agency of our Being. It was present in the times of slavery and it is present in every oppressive system. It seems it was glorified and comingled with dignity and independence during the Nixon era, where they began to define our joys for us in jobs and working, independence as the source of dignity, further dismantling the BIPOC connection with Being, Nature, and Spirit, and keeping one busy in activity and endless striving. It would catapult up to now, where too much too fast is the norm while rest and reflection are a death. The practice here is to find a place of gratitude; to be with what is and to notice it with your whole body. It is when we allow this level of noticings that we can connect with the primordial nature of everything. Our nature is connected with all there is.

The Everyday

The year 2020 showed us that in order to make collective change, we have to make it an individual daily practice or ritual. We have been good about being busy and engaged in several different activities, but this approach has left us tired and discursive about what is needed. These three doors and their practice offer the opportunity to approach what is needed with a mind that is clear and stable so that our action is effective and expansive enough to hold both the relative truth of the moment and also the absolute interconnectedness of all things. I invite you to listen to Stevie Wonder's song "As." Be inspired to love ourselves just as absolutely and expansively.

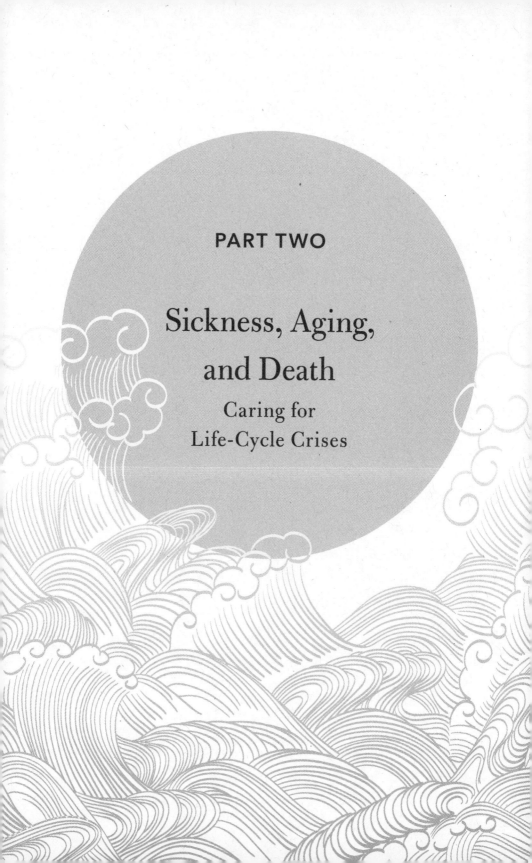

PART TWO

Sickness, Aging, and Death

Caring for Life-Cycle Crises

9

STAYING COOL DURING A CODE BLUE

Caring for a Distressed Fiancée

Manling Lim

D uring my clinical pastoral education residency to train as a chaplain, I worked at a hospital and Level 1 trauma center in North Carolina. In a trauma center, "code blue," which refers to the medical emergency in which a patient is in cardiopulmonary arrest, was not an uncommon alert to hear. When I first started working there, though, they induced significant anxiety in me. The following story, however, comes from a time when I began a transition in my reaction toward focusing on what I *can* do (caring for the people in front of me) while accepting what was beyond my control (saving a person's life). This shift helped deepen my ministry of presence with the patients and led me to integrate my Buddhist tradition more deeply into care for people's needs.

Accompanying a Distressed Fiancée

During my overnight on-call shift, I received a brief phone call from a staff member asking me to be with the wife of a patient who was brought to the hospital's catheterization lab. Natalie's fiancé was taken in during a heart attack and she was outside the room, sitting by herself. When I arrived, I could see a middle-aged woman in a green hoodie standing in the hallway, weeping and covering her mouth with one hand. I introduced myself, and then a staff member who accompanied her showed us to the small physician consultation room nearby before leaving us alone to talk. I sat next to Natalie on the couch in the room.

"Can you tell me what happened?"

"He passed out."

"I just want to make sure you know that they didn't call me because something bad will happen. They just wanted to give you some support."

"I just want," she struggled to say, "Danny to be OK."

"What's your relationship?"

"I'm his fiancée."

"Oh, I can't imagine how hard this must be for you."

"I don't want to lose him. I just don't want to lose him. I can't . . ." She then buried her face in her hands while adding, "My ex-husband died the same way."

We sat in some silence when she needed to, but I gradually heard some of the story about her ex-husband's condition and passing. I also learned that, although her children played a critical role in helping her through that grief, they were living on the other side of the country, thousands of miles away. She felt alone in this new city, now probably more than ever. I listened to her stories of other family members passing and how that was affecting her in this moment, but also just stayed by her in silence at times. I had gradually become more comfortable with this "ministry of presence" through the experience of chaplaincy, when just being there with another felt more important than any words could express.

I went to get some water for her after she requested it, but on my way back, I heard a code blue being called overhead from the cath lab. I tried to check to see if I could get any brief updates on Danny's status, but to no avail. I felt a deep anxiety arising in me, but tried to notice it and calm back down, both for my own sake and for Natalie. When I returned to the room, the alarm was still on and Natalie was clearly deeply nervous. I poured her water.

"Is it him?" she asked anxiously.

"Sorry," I replied, "I tried to find out, but I couldn't get any details."

After a pause in silence, the alarm was turned off and we continued to sit in silence.

"It feels like an eternity," she suddenly said, while looking up at me.

"It is a long wait," I said.

She struggled to reply. "Did . . . did he die?"

"Usually, doctors will come and inform family members if that happens, but no doctor has come yet."

She looked back up at me anxiously and then suddenly and eagerly asked, "Can we pray?"

"Sure, let's pray together," I replied, as reassuringly as I could, though internally I noticed anxiety still in me. "Holy One, thank you for your presence. Help us feel your presence even more during this wait and give us peace. We sincerely pray that with all the good things he has done, Danny can make it through these trying times. In your name, Amen."

"Thank you," she said. "How do you think he is right now?"

I told her that doctors here were good with giving important updates, but that I would go and check if she wanted me to.

I was able to find out that doctors had only just opened a vessel near Danny's heart and were waiting a few minutes to proceed with the next steps. However, Danny was still alive. I updated Natalie about the status as soon as I returned to her side. After a little pause, I mentioned there was a cafeteria nearby if she needed anything. She touched her chest and said she felt like throwing up.

"Let's go back into the consultation room and sit down. Take a few deep breaths." I helped guide her through several deep breaths, but she still seemed extremely anxious with her mind on Danny. "Have you ever heard of a finger labyrinth? I have one with me." She took glasses out of her handbag while I rummaged through papers in a folder to pull it out. I gave her some basic instructions on how to trace her finger through. A labyrinth is an ancient technique used by different cultures and religions for meditation and prayer. The participants follow a meandering path from the outside of the labyrinth to the center and then back out on the same path. A finger labyrinth is a portable version, and users trace the labyrinth from the nondominant hand. This directs the mind to focus on simply following the pattern and quiets other thought processes, giving rise to a sense of peacefulness. I previously introduced the finger labyrinth to patients and families who were waiting for updates or making a decision, and they appreciated it, so I thought it would be a nice distraction for Natalie as she anxiously waited for updates.

While she focused on "walking" the labyrinth, two doctors came into the room with updates.

"He is alive. He is still quite ill. But we are going to continue doing our best in taking care of him, OK?" Natalie seemed calmer, and called Danny's daughter, who was on her way to the hospital, to share this update with her.

I continued to sit with Natalie for a while longer, before asking her permission to leave to get ready for other patients, but provided my contact information in the hospital in case she needed me.

Practices and Lessons in Buddhist Chaplaincy

Although I am a dedicated Buddhist practitioner, Natalie was not and never inquired about my religious background. Of course, I never tried to push my Buddhist viewpoints onto her; yet my Buddhist background helped inform my interactions with her and helped establish chaplaincy practices that I found beneficial to develop from there on. In this section, I will discuss four such ways that I applied my spiritual background as a Buddhist in this case, which have also more generally benefited my own personal chaplaincy practice.

1. **Centering and Grounding:** Up until the visit with Natalie, I had been practicing noticing my bodily sensations to become more self-aware. The method I used to center and ground myself was to focus on my in-and-out breaths. Through my practice, I had gradually cultivated some level of sensitivity to the texture and rhythm of my breathing in my own contemplative time outside work. Becoming aware of my breathing served as an anchor I was grateful for as I stepped into a whirlwind of dealing with people in crisis situations on the job.

More importantly, the aforementioned practice served as a base that helped me access deeper calm than I would have probably been able to within very short periods of practice between patient visits. I was then able to develop a whole-body awareness within the clinical setting so that, even if I lost my focus of my in-and-out breaths, I could maintain my internal balance to a degree. I developed this whole-body awareness with the perception of being a "mobile home" through which I could rest and recharge myself anywhere I go.

I approached my patient visits with a similar intention and awareness as I did for sitting meditation at home, using breath as a focal point as described above. I also treated the walks from one patient room to the next as a form of walking meditation to release myself from the thoughts and feelings from previous visits. These practices helped me to become more mindful of my mental, emotional, and physical states and to stay centered and grounded amid chaos.

2. **Trusting My Presence:** I trusted that simply showing up to be with the fiancée during a terrible night of her life was already part of the act of caring. Through more experience with chaplaincy, I became comfortable with *doing* little, shifted the emphasis to the *being* with the patient. I knew that one way to help the fiancée get through this time was to model a calming presence rather than trying to "fix" anything about her. Such a desire to fix others tended to arise from my own anxiety, an important personal realization that led me to *be* with my patients as they were in a way that was more deeply aware.

This grew out of my personal definition of ministry: to bring peace and security to other living beings through goodwill, compassion, empathetic joy, and equanimity (the four *brahmavihārās*). Goodwill is a wish for true and sustainable happiness, both for me and for others. Compassion is a wish for all beings to be free from stress and pain. Empathetic joy is a wish that other living beings will not lose the happiness they've found. Equanimity is an attitude to keep my mind calm and balanced when there is nothing I can do to help alleviate others' suffering.

In the function of spiritual care, these sublime attitudes help me hold space for people in their times of crisis and distress. I practice staying grounded when listening to other people's stories so that they feel seen and heard. I use these attitudes to try and cultivate a calming and soothing energy, in the hope that such energy may also provide comfort to people I care for and help them connect with their own spiritual resources.

For example, I applied this practice during one of my visits with a patient who had an argument with a staff member and was verbally abusive toward a few nurses. The patient talked about his frustration regarding his illness and lengthy hospitalization, and did not show any obvious signs of calming down by the end of my visit. But I listened to him and maintained my goodwill and compassion, wishing that he could find some peace despite his illness and be free from his mental pain. The next day, however, he told me that he apologized to the nurses and expressed his appreciation for their care. This experience affirmed my belief that goodwill and compassion can be felt by other living beings as long as they are receptive to it. It may not happen instantly and we may never know the full affects our attitudes have, but that doesn't mean we should stop. I believe these attitudes are ultimately beneficial to both the provider and recipient of care.

3. **Listening Skills:** Listening is one of the most important skills in chaplaincy and I think the brahmavihārās are also very applicable in cultivating deeper listening. The challenge in listening deeply to others lies in being present with the feelings underneath. During the first half of my chaplaincy residency, I intentionally worked on dealing with my own negative feelings and being better attuned to my emotions and those of others. Developing heart qualities through the cultivation of the brahmavihārās described above expanded my capacity to care and connect with others, and led to a better ability to listen to all the subtle cues that people provide in communication. For example, being equanimous about difficult feelings arising in me keeps me from shutting down while listening to others as they express strenuous emotions.

Being emotionally attuned to others helps me hear deeper layers of emotions that might be expressed either verbally or nonverbally. Working on this helped me to hear the layers of fear and grief in Natalie's statement, "I'm just tired of losing people." It helped me hear both her vulnerability and hope in her request to pray together.

The listening skills during crisis care are built on the listening skills I used in daily visits. I usually adopt the relational-cultural theory, which posits that we grow through and toward relationships throughout our lives and that growth-fostering relationships are the source of meaning and empowerment. I seek to relate to my patients as fellow human beings with the warmth of connection and stay emotionally open and authentic to facilitate a "movement in relationship." In this way, the patient "has the very valuable chance to know that her thoughts and feelings do reach another person, do matter, and can be part of a mutual experience."[1]

4. **Spiritual Assessment:** Spiritual assessment is an important aspect of care, involving an in-depth exploration of patients' spiritual hopes, concerns, and needs, which can help in some factors of determining treatment plans and the ways in which care providers engage the patient. The model I used with Natalie in the example above was spiritual distress assessment tool (SDAT). The

hypothesis was that spiritual distress arises from unmet spiritual needs. In this model, spirituality is defined as a multidimensional concept that includes four dimensions: meaning, transcendence, values, and psychosocial identity. The meaning dimension deals with how much the overall life balance of a patient is disturbed. The transcendence dimension focuses on a patient's need to be connected with the personal existential anchor and how their spirituality or faith is challenged by what's happening to them. The values dimension addresses a patient's need to understand and be involved in caregivers' decisions and actions. The psychosocial identity represents an individual's need to maintain identity (to be loved, listened to, have a positive self-image, and so on).

Natalie's physical reaction while waiting to hear about her fiancée included nausea, which hinted to me the degree of disturbance to her overall sense of life balance. Yet her request for prayer indicated that she was still connected with her personal existential anchor. Her patience in waiting for updates, despite her worry, showed that her need to understand the caregivers' actions was met. How she talked to her family on the phone calls implied that her need to maintain identity was also met.

On the whole, however, I could see Natalie was very overwhelmed by the situation and the conditions suggested that she could benefit from grounding herself at that moment. Therefore, I focused my intervention on trying to aid her overall sense of life balance and adopted a phenomenological approach to help her feel grounded in the here and now. I used my experience in integrative healing modalities to introduce her to both simple breathing techniques and a finger labyrinth that both seemed to fit within her spiritual attenuation. Even if my approach bore some of my own Buddhist practice and background, it was adapted in a way to fit her and that particular moment. Fortunately, she responded well to these areas and seemed to calm down enough to maintain the composure she needed for her own psychological well-being and for communication on the phone with her relatives.

Conclusions

The visit with Natalie affirmed the importance of an old saying for me: "put on your own oxygen mask before helping others with their masks." I think this is all the more important when helping those in crisis situations. I made sure that I was grounded before entering the room and I tried to continue taking care of myself as I was trying to take care of the distraught fiancée. I was watching my energy level, since I had worked on the day shift and there was a night shift scheduled ahead. I tried not to overextend myself and replenished my own energy while I sat with her in silence. I also used the act of getting water for her as an opportunity to partially disconnect from the situation; this gave me a short break to check in with myself more fully and ensure I was properly grounded. I learned from this visit that these little acts of self-care were not selfish but necessary for me to provide quality care for the patients and sustain my own well-being in the process.

The connection between the caregiver and the care seeker itself can be healing during times of crisis. It's also an important competency to build connection with care seekers from diverse cultural and religious backgrounds—and to try to find those common grounds and connecting points relatively quickly within what can be brief encounters. No matter who is in front of us, it is our job to provide presence and see their own needs from their spiritual ground. The previously mentioned relational-cultural theory has something to offer in this aspect. As Maureen Walker wrote,

> empathy is more than a feeling. It is a multidimensional portal to expanded possibility. . . . Respect is foundational to empathy. Without it, we are unable to open ourselves to the different-ness and the complexity we encounter in ourselves and in others. It is openness to difference that allows our relational frames, our deep structured narrative about power to shift.[2]

By grounding ourselves, trusting our presence, listening deeply to others, and assessing our own needs, we would find it easier to be there for others—even in the context of a code blue.

10

A BUDDHIST
CHAPLAIN'S PRAYER

Anna Gagnon

In my work as a hospital chaplain, I often minister to people in times of spiritual and emotional distress. I might be asked to speak with a patient hours before they undergo a life-threatening surgery, or perhaps just after they receive news of a troubling diagnosis. I might sit with a family member who is considering forgoing further treatment for a loved one, their heart conflicted about accepting hospice. I might spend time holding a young child's hand as she wakes up after a car accident and finds herself alone in the emergency room. The circumstances are always different but the suffering is uniquely real.

Among the many interventions I use in hospital ministry, enabling patients and family members to connect with their *spiritual practices* is one of the most important ways I can support their coping. Spiritual practices are as diverse as the patients I serve: scripture reading, breath work, singing, meditation, silent reflection, chanting, ritualizing, visualization, physical movement, or devotional worship. In a moment of anguish or uncertainty, such practices can be a lifeline. They can soothe and comfort us, feed and strengthen us spiritually. Spiritual practices can move our faith out of abstraction and into the reality of life here and now. They can help bring what is sacred close again, when we need it most.

Of all the spiritual practices I encounter in ministry, prayer is by far the most prevalent. Over the years, I have been honored to pray with individuals from almost every major religion, along with countless others who did not adhere to traditional religious frameworks. Often, I am a supportive participant in another person's act of prayer. I kneel down next to a young mother at her son's bedside. She reaches over to take my hand and begins to pray in her native language. Here, I am an honored guest, humbled to be brought into her world. Other times, I am the leader of prayer. I put voice to my patients' petitions and intentions; help them navigate the language of their heart. When I lead, I do my best to honor each person's unique style of prayer—in a way that is both respectful of their tradition and authentic to myself. And finally, there are times when I am neither leader nor participant; times when I use my pastoral authority to create the space for prayer. With my words or with my silence, I invite a shift from speaking about prayer in the abstract and into a moment of authentic engagement. I make a safe and supportive container for practice to begin.

Clara is weeping quietly on the bed in front of me. She came into the hospital after falling on an icy patch in her driveway. But this is not why she is crying. While recovering from her injuries, two potentially lethal aneurysms were discovered on a CT scan. Doctors theorize that Clara has probably had these aneurysms for years. Indeed, they could have easily killed her at any time. As I sit down beside her, Clara begins to tell me what it is like to have received this news, to have been given such a real sense of her own mortality: "I keep thinking back on all the moments I could have died . . . all the time that could have been lost."

In Buddhist terms, Clara has touched the two sides of impermanence. She has felt both the *fragility* and the *preciousness* of life. Such an encounter has offered her a momentary *bardo,* a period of time in which Clara's habitual responses have been put on hold. She is suddenly free to look upon her life with fresh eyes. Ripe for meaning-making and reflection, Clara tells me that she is sure God has intervened to renew her dwindling faith. "Whether I die tomorrow in surgery or not, I know now that God is very real. He never left me. *I left Him.*"

Because I am the hospital chaplain, it is clear that Clara has invited me into her room to bear witness to her testimony and hear the central longing of her heart. Above all, Clara wishes to renew her connection with God. "I used to have a very personal relationship with God, but all that changed after the death of my son. . . . Now I want it back again. I want God back in my life." Clara reflects on all the anger and resentment she once carried, the very real shadows of her grief. She speaks of bitterness and betrayal, years of heartache, but always in the past tense. A quiet sadness fills her voice now.

I invite Clara to describe what her relationship with God *felt* like in her heart and body. She whispers: "I could feel it in the morning. He was the first thing I thought about when I woke up ... and the last thing at night. It brought me such ... well, it brought me joy. ... I used to tell Him everything." After a long silence, I ask Clara if she would like to try talking to God *right now*. She nods, and there is another hesitant pause. Then Clara begins to pray, and the passion of her words catches me off guard. Her prayer is candid and direct, stripped of all pretense. The weight of it slowly fills the room. Clara speaks of regret and asks for forgiveness. She talks of gratitude and awe, fear and relief. It is a powerful and revealing moment, and for a long time, I am simply spellbound. I am wrapped in this person's intimate and sincere efforts to connect both with herself and with her God.

Then I hear a thought—a question, really—whispering in the back of my mind. It won't let me be: *And what do you believe is happening here, Anna? Who or what is this person talking to—to God? To herself? To the part of herself that is God? How would you explain this moment?*

As a young child in a Catholic family, I prayed often and with fervor. I loved attending church, especially the moments when the priest would grow quiet and allow the congregants to silently lift up their petitions and inner thoughts. A moment of deep listening. I never really stopped praying, even when I became a Buddhist at nineteen. Though it's true that the act of prayer was slowly usurped in my heart by meditation. It was only after a master's degree in Buddhism, and years of training as a Buddhist chaplain, that I realized how important it was for me to revisit my understanding of prayer. What did it mean for me to pray? It was Clara, and patients like her, who brought the gravity of such questions to the forefront.

For a nontheistic tradition, one could say that the divisions of Buddhism are littered with gods. Tibetan Buddhism, in particular, uses hundreds of images of gods, goddesses, *dakinis,* and bodhisattvas in visualization practices. The difference being that such conceptions of the divine are never to be understood as something solid, permanent, or most importantly, outside oneself. Indeed, such practices often culminate in the visualization of oneself *as* the godhead—the self-manifestation of the mudra and the mandala within the immediacy of one's own experience.

When I bow in front of an altar with such images, I am bowing to the same capacity within my own mind. I am bowing to the intention—the aspiration—that I can transcend the illusion of separateness and realize my own innate potential for complete and utter liberation. In the Theravāda traditions of Southeast Asia, the symbol of the lotus flower is often used when bowing. If you have ever seen a lotus bud, two hands coming together look a bit like it. And of course, the lotus flower can rise up and bloom in even the dirtiest and murkiest of swamps. It can be born fresh and pure in the harshest of environments. In one temple, I was taught to bow and say: "A lotus flower for you, future Buddha," honoring the sacredness of the one who stood before me. In other words, regardless of the harshness or mire of the current suffering, there is always the possibility of perfect and complete enlightenment around every corner. It is the face of God, the face of Jesus, the way of Buddha, in each person I meet: "A lotus flower for you, future Buddha." In the Zen tradition of Japan, *no separation* is often emphasized in the act of bowing. The word *gasshō* is Japanese for "to place the two palms together." It represents two hands, two sides, two opposites becoming one. Self and other—the bower and the one being bowed to—are not so far apart in this act. I bow to you, Buddha. I take refuge in you, and doing so, you take refuge in me: two becoming one.

Of course, such insights rest on the Doctrine of the Two Truths, a foundational teaching that can be found in all divisions of Buddhism. While this doctrine only appears on the periphery of the Nikāya traditions, it plays a foundational role in Mahāyāna Buddhism and cannot be emphasized enough. To summarize, the doctrine states that, in every context, individuals may either recognize relative truth or absolute truth. Legendary Buddhist scholar Chandrakīrti taught that relative truth is associated with the false seeing of worldly beings. It is how we conventionally experience our daily life. It is an understanding imbedded in samsara and marred by ignorance and craving. In contrast, ultimate truth represents the genuine seeing of a Buddha. It is the same circumstance experienced through the eyes of an enlightened mind. This is the manifestation of nirvana. In this way, it is important to understand that the two truths do not refer to two entirely separate realms of existence, but simply two different modes of perception. They identify an epistemological distinction, not an ontological one.[1] What is more, it is essential to understand that ultimate truth is neither the cause nor the result of anything else; it simply *is.* As my Tibetan teacher says: "Ultimate truth is the very intimate and real experience of 'suchness'; life as it is." It may be tempting to disregard relative truth as mere confusion and to believe that it carries no validity or importance. However, relative truth is absolutely essential to the Buddhist path. In many ways, it is the path. It is the method by which we gain experience of ultimate reality. It shows us the places where our craving for life as we wish it to be rubs up against life as it is. In the end, recognition of both truths is necessary for liberation.

But what does all of this have to do with Clara and the vividness of her yearnings and prayer? In his book *The Energy of Prayer,* Thich Nhat Hanh addresses five central questions about the act of worship and prayer. The most central inquiry, the one on which all the others rest, is: *"Who is the person to whom I pray?"* Indeed, it is very similar to the question that came to me during my visit with Clara. Like me, Thich Nhat Hanh returns to the famous Buddhist mantra: "The one who bows and the one who is bowed to are both, by nature, empty." Emptiness, of course, does not mean a state of lack or nothingness. Quite the contrary, emptiness refers to *being empty of a separate self,* and in fact, *being full of all that is*—interdependence. In the end, this mantra is about reexamining the fragile boundary between self and other, self and God. Describing prayer as a type of spiritual practice, Hanh concludes:

> When we pray in Buddhism, we are praying both to ourselves and to what is outside of ourselves; there is no distinction. If, in truth, we are practicing, then we can see that we also have the same substance of love, mindfulness, and understanding as all the great beings. God and we are of the same substance. Between God and us there is no discrimination, no separation.[2]

In prayer, I practice manifesting the experience of ultimate truth, the truth of no separation. I practice the outlook of the enlightened mind. I call out to the presence of love and compassion, wisdom and insight that resides in this world. So doing, I connect to that same presence within myself.

Does intercessory prayer work? Can prayer change cause and effect, the results of our karmic actions? If we understand enlightenment as a radical shift in perspective, then I believe it can. I can change the course of my life and the lives of others by working to manifest such divinity here and now. I pray for God's love with my patients, and so doing, I make an aspiration to *feel* loved, and to bring that love into the hospital room. I call out to God to enter my life and the lives of my patients, and so doing, I begin to make space for God here and now. I begin to connect with the God that is already within me, waiting to bloom and blossom at any moment. As Thich Nhat Hanh tells us: *we practice praying both to ourselves and to what is outside of ourselves; there is no distinction.*

Christian theologian C. S. Lewis wrote: "I don't pray to change God's mind, I pray to change my mind. I pray because I can't help myself, because I am helpless. I pray because the need just flows out of me all the time—waking and sleeping." In the face of our limits and helplessness, in the face of old age, sickness, and death, we call out in prayer. But it is not God's mind that is changed by such cries; it is our own. It is the God within us blooming with the aspiration to trust and accept life as it is.

Prayer changes life at its very foundation because it changes the way we perceive it.

YOUR CHAPLAIN

At the death of your sister,
You gave me two maps of Klickitat County.
I, a stranger, made real only because of the once dying body that
Stood lying on the plastic bed in front of us—a body
Long gone gray around the tubing that pierced it.

You gave me these maps without shame
Without irony
With an almost childish eagerness
Quickly wanting to open the folds and feathers of their accordion nature
Out over the sheet that covered your sister's legs.
Landscape on top of landscape, veins on top of veins
The red and blue lines falling over the edge of the mattress.

Here, you point, here is the dark hillside where we played as children.
The place she parked her trailer after the divorce.
The gap where she often crossed the river with her dog.

I, feeling awkward and awed by the way your grief chose to
Bleed at that moment, was left speechless.
So I put my hands on the map with you.

Momentarily feeling the shape of the person beneath it
The stiff bend of a knee, a furrowed hand

And I thought
it was really three maps we were tracing here.
One over the land, one over time,
One over the flesh of death—the fingers of loss
already beginning to untie you from this, your sister's body.

I sit beside you.
Having followed along the narrows, you grow quiet;
Begin to collect the maps up into themselves
Their pleats hinging closed. Your grief, turning its face from me.
Something unseen has tracked and found itself. Been reconciled.
Though I know not what.

At your insistence, I take the maps home with me
Unsure of what to do with them.
But then you will have them, you say,
If you ever decide to go to Klickitat County.
You could visit these places.
I know she would have liked that.

11

MAKING FRIENDS WITH THE ANEURYSM IN MY BRAIN

Noel Alumit

I was having problems speaking. My tongue felt lazy, like part of it was paralyzed. A friend said I should look into it. After all, my livelihood revolves around me speaking. I lecture, I facilitate meditation groups, I perform. Speaking is important to me.

I called the advice nurse on a Tuesday—it was a beautiful spring day in Los Angeles. The sky was blue, the air was clear. I planned a bike ride in the afternoon. I thought the nurse might set up an appointment for me to come in the next few days because, surely, it couldn't be that serious. The advice nurse suggested I come in immediately because I might be having a stroke. A stroke? Strokes run in my family. An aunt had a stroke at fifty-two—oh, my God, I'm fifty-two!

I went to the ER. They had to do a CT scan.

Roberto, the nurse who took care of me before the scan, was jovial and friendly. He said, "How are you doing today?"

"I'm in the ER, how do you think I'm doing?" I joked.

He laughed and said, "Hopefully, this won't be too bad."

The CT scan was performed and, afterward, Roberto was quiet.

"I'll take you back to your room," he said. I noted his change in tone, from friendly to serious.

"You're not having a stroke," said Dr. Singh, the ER doctor.

I had a fistula, or more simply, the nerves in my brain were not properly wired. They needed to fix it, but it wasn't life threatening.

Good, I thought. No problem.

"We found something else in your CT scan," he said.

He performed some coordination tests to check my motor skills. Another doctor entered: Dr. Chan, a neurologist.

"We found something in your X-ray," Dr. Chan said. "We found an aneurysm in your brain. An aneurysm is a nerve blockage that builds and fills like a balloon. If it bursts, it could be fatal or cause severe neurological damage."

I knew someone who suffered an aneurysm. She was a comedian. She became permanently brain damaged and lost her ability to speak. Her livelihood gone.

The singer Laura Branigan died of it. She complained of headaches, went to bed, and never woke up.

Dr. Chan also checked my motor skills, asking me to press his hands with my hands and pull on his fingers. Then he asked, "What year is it?"

"2020."

"Where are you?"

"I'm in the ER at Kaiser."

He wanted to make sure I could make sense of my surroundings.

"We're going to schedule more tests," he said.

Wait. I was supposed to be on my bike, enjoying this beautiful spring day. I wasn't supposed to be in an ER and certainly wasn't supposed to have an aneurysm in my brain.

I'm a Buddhist. This was impermanence. Things change so quickly. I went from planning a bike ride to getting scheduled for an MRI and a cranial angiogram. As for my fistula, the nerves causing my lazy tongue, I also had consultations about that. The best course of action was radiation.

"You might lose some hair," a doctor said, "but it should grow back."

Oh, man, you mean in addition to worrying about an aneurysm, I have to think about the side effects of radiation treatment? It was the best viable option. It was the least invasive and the least risky. The other options could have risked me losing the use of one side of my face.

Impermanence. Damn it.

Suddenly, I was directionless, vulnerable, even grief-stricken over the kind of life I thought I was supposed to have and the one I might have. I recalled the mustard seed story. It was the tale of Kisa Gotami in the Therīgāthā, which contains the stories of the first Buddhist nuns.

Kisa Gotami's child had died. She went to the Buddha for help. The Buddha said he could help her but she must find a mustard seed and return it to the Buddha. There was a caveat. The mustard seed could not come from a home that had experienced grief.

Kisa Gotami went from house to house looking for a home that hadn't known this kind of sorrow. She discovered that every home she'd visited had known this kind of pain. Kisa Gotami's story ends like this. After finding no house that was free of grief and pain, she thought:

"This is the way it will be in the entire city.

"By means of the Buddha's compassion for my welfare, this will be what is seen."

And having gained a sense of spiritual urgency from that, she went out and covered her son in the charnel ground.

She uttered this verse:

It's not just a truth for one village or town,
Nor is it a truth for a single family.
But for every world settled by gods [and humans]
This indeed is what is true—impermanence.

And so saying, she went into the presence of the Buddha.
Then the Buddha said to her,
"Have you obtained, Gotami, the mustard seed?"
"Finished, sir, is the matter of the mustard seed," she said.
"You have indeed restored me."

And the Buddha uttered this verse:
A person with a mind that clings,
Deranged, to children or possessions,
Is swept away by death that comes—
Like mighty flood to sleeping town.

At the conclusion of this verse, confirmed in the fruit of stream-entry, she asked the Buddha [for permission] to go forth [into the holy life]. The Buddha allowed her to go forth. She gave homage to the Buddha by bowing three times, went to join the community of nuns, and having gone forth, received her ordination.

It was not long before, through the doing of deeds with careful attention, she caused her insight to grow, and she became an arahant . . . a truly free person who experienced nirvana.[1]

•

Buddhist scholar Bhikkhu Bodhi explained,

> For suffering to give birth to a genuine spiritual search, it must amount to more than something passively received from without. It has to trigger an inner realization, a perception which pierces through the facile complacency of our usual encounter with the world to glimpse the insecurity perpetually gaping underfoot.[2]

That last phrase resonates with me: "the insecurity perpetually gaping underfoot . . ."

I should not cling to what I think life is supposed to be. Buddha's words are not meant to be pessimistic or morbid. Rather, we're asking to be open to surprises. And not all surprises are bad.

Not clinging means being open to all possibilities, including good ones. Through all of this, I found out that I received a grant that will help me develop a novel I'd been thinking about. The grant will relieve some financial pressure. I found friends and family willing to support me through this time, affirming my choices in the community I choose to be in. And, lastly, this experience affirms Buddhism as a foundation for my life.

Finding out I had an aneurysm will keep me alert. It's small now. I'll have it monitored annually to see if it grows. I've been warned: If I have severe headaches, don't hesitate to go to the ER.

I'd made friends with my aneurysm—I call her Annie. I say, "Hi, Annie, I'll take good care of me—lower my blood pressure—so it won't exacerbate your growth." I'll be good to Annie if she'll be good to me.

There are times when I get migraines and I wonder if this is *it!* Will this turn into the forewarned headache that might end my life or leave me permanently disabled?

Maybe.

Or maybe not.

The *Game of Thrones* actress Emilia Clarke had two aneurysms, but they caught them early. President Joe Biden also had aneurysms but fortunately survived them. In both cases, much suffering was caused as both endured physical and emotional pain. This included enduring surgery on one of the most delicate parts of the body—the brain.

Others have lived their entire lives without an aneurysm causing any harm.

I don't know which one will be me. I don't know if I will be randomly hit by a car or caught in a mass shooting. I simply don't know.

With that sentiment, I repeat Kisa Gotami's words to the Buddha: You have indeed restored me.

12

A BUDDHIST COUNSELING APPROACH FOR ADVANCED CANCER

Kin Cheung (George) Lee, PhD

Crisis is a natural part of life. According to Albert R. Roberts, a psychological definition of crisis is "an acute disruption of psychological homeostasis in which one's usual coping mechanisms fail, and there exists evidence of distress and functional impairment."[1] Separation from loved ones, undesirable events and people, sickness, aging, and dying are some of the classifications of suffering *(dukkha)* in Buddhism as well as common crisis-inducing events in the contemporary world. Among these categories of suffering, any endangerment to bodily integrity is one of the most challenging crises to manage. In particular, there were 17 million new cases of cancer worldwide with 9.6 million cancer deaths in 2018. There will be an estimated 27.5 million new cases of cancer each year by 2040. Advanced cancer, a chronic condition with limited life prognosis, may be ubiquitous, unpredictable, and unavoidable, and in turn, it is time to consider the importance of crisis care while attending to such patients.

Assisting a person with cancer, who is going through the process of sickness and dying, to arrive at a simple moment of peace and understanding is an invaluable gift that a Buddhist chaplain or other care provider can offer. At such a critical time, it would be ideal for a Buddhist patient to be comforted by a chaplain of the same faith. For Buddhist patients, the Buddhist chaplaincy provides a faith companion for spiritual care, for developing a new and more positive understanding of life in the moments before death, for consoling their fears, processing other negative emotions, and supporting family members through grief and loss. However, there has been a lack of resources to guide people in providing Buddhist care for this particular group.

In professional psychology, there are several conceptual frameworks developed to facilitate the work of social workers, psychologists, and other mental health professionals providing services to cancer patients. For example, Jevne, Nekolaichuk, and Williamson proposed a patient-centered counseling model within the context of cancer that is designed as a problem-solving approach with a strong emphasis on understanding the client's worldview as well as their experiences with the illness.[2] This model also focuses on enhancing hope and deepening commitment. Moreover, knowing that family members of a cancer patient can also suffer from tremendous stress, there are systemic approaches for cancer patients. Sherman and Simonton delineated clinical issues and considerations in providing family therapy within the context of cancer.[3]

Particularly, there are specific treatment directions to provide education and support, enhance communication, promote positive structural changes in the family dynamic, construct shared meaning, and confront mortality in the family system. Although these models can be effective for certain populations and cultures, most of them were developed from Western Judeo-Christian backgrounds and many models do not have an emphasis on spirituality and religiosity. In response, Raweewan Pilaikiat et al. proposed a Buddhist spiritual care conceptual model that places a strong focus on patients' spirituality.[4] The model provides a strong conceptual framework where there has not been specific treatment guidelines, considerations, and examples for care providers. Taken together, the resources for Buddhist care providers are a smattering compared to that in professional psychology. The traditional Western models, including the secularization of mindfulness-based interventions, may not be culturally congruent to patients with Buddhist affiliations, and it is essential to provide more pragmatic resources for frontline Buddhist spiritual care providers.

In response to the rising criticisms of the Western application of mindfulness, some scholars have begun to develop treatment models and interventions based on traditional Buddhist teaching. Among those treatment models, this chapter will introduce the author's model of Buddhist counseling to discuss considerations and interventions for individuals in crises to facilitate the work of Buddhist chaplains, Buddhist counselors, and other mental health and well-being professionals interested in adopting a Buddhist approach to advanced cancer.[5]

The Note, Know, Choose Model:
A Brief Introduction

As one of the Buddhist counseling models, the Note, Know, Choose approach reflects the essence of mental processes and provides the main ingredients for therapeutic change in action terms.[6] Different from many psychotherapies or counseling models, Note, Know, Choose is a flexible framework that can include a range of mental activities, ranging from a moment of mindfulness to a full-blown treatment process. The Note, Know, Choose model uses an iterative three-phase process with interventions that (a) raise clients' ability to concentrate, (b) increase clients' insight into the causes of their suffering, and (c) reveal ways to reduce suffering and strengthen clients' ability to make better decisions at every moment. The ideal state of mind comprises (a) stillness and peace to note mental events; (b) discernment to know how these events arise and cease and how they increase or reduce suffering; and (c) mindfulness to deliberatively choose to think, act, or speak in ways that result in the least amount of suffering. In this model, "choose" refers to volition, a subtle mental decision that fuels mental and bodily actions. Choosing between either giving in to previous negative patterns or making a change in those patterns is perhaps the most crucial starting point. It is a continuous volition to foster and sustain a wholesome state of mind.

The Note, Know, Choose Model
for Chronic Illness

Cancer is one of the scariest illnesses in present-day life. Being diagnosed with cancer frequently leads to emotional turmoil, including shock, fear for the future, worries about treatment, anger and resentment ("Why me?"), sadness, and hopelessness.[7] Moreover, cancer patients have to cope with various physical symptoms such as pain, appetite loss, fatigue, and the multiple side effects of surgery, chemotherapy, radiotherapy, and other medical procedures. Many cancer patients reported a loss of control over life, forced changes in roles, concern for the psychological distress of family and loved ones, and heightened levels of anxiety and depression.[8]

There are many forms of advanced cancer, and each patient has a unique experience due to their background. Therefore, the first consideration for Buddhist care providers is to maintain an open attitude to understand each patient according to their gender, class, culture, diagnosis, bodily function, treatment, and other specific conditions. This process also requires flexibility and creativity to adapt a chaplain's Buddhist knowledge and counseling skills to fit the patient's idiosyncratic needs. As the first step to cultivate openness, flexibility, and creativity, Buddhist chaplains should understand the importance of their mind and presence as therapeutic tools for patients.

Mind Preparation

The competency to provide spiritual care is directly proportionate to the Buddhist chaplain's level of mental cultivation. In particular, a highly cultivated Buddhist chaplain with a natural presence of compassion and loving-kindness is likely to offer warmth and trust in the therapeutic process. The chaplain's deep listening also dissolves the client's sorrows and lamentations, and the chaplain can understand clients' causes of suffering based on their direct experiences with cultivation. Moreover, cultivated Buddhist chaplains should have developed a routine of spiritual practices as a self-care method and an ongoing pursuit for liberation that allows them to rejuvenate after caring for clients and progressively reducing their suffering. For these reasons, Buddhist chaplains or others working with cancer patients can benefit from developing specific habits of cultivation to enhance their competency. This chapter provides several suggestions for practice.

- Develop a daily mindfulness practice and commit to immersing yourself fully in this practice without distractions.

- Regularly practice loving-kindness meditation and radiating compassion to yourself, the cancer patients under your care, and all patients who have cancer.

- Get to know your limits so that you know when to consult, rest, or get help.

- Regularly contemplate on your three poisons (greed, aversions, ignorance) related to your work. Care providers can use the following sets
  of questions for reflection to understand potential hindrances to your
  spiritual care:

  1. **Contemplation on ignorance:** What is my attitude toward cancer?
     What stereotypes do I associate with cancer? What do I know about
     my patient's cancer and suffering, and what do I not know? What is
     my personal experience with cancer, and how does it help or interfere
     with my competency to provide care?

  2. **Contemplation on greed:** What do I hope to achieve in my time
     with this patient? What would be in the best interest of this patient?
     Am I expecting something out of my control?

  3. **Contemplation on aversion:** What makes me uncomfortable,
     afraid, frustrated, or resistant in the process? What are the inner
     voices associated with these feelings?

These practices and contemplations are likely to help care providers prevent
burnout and strengthen their therapeutic presence to attend to cancer patients.

Note

The initial phase, Note, has the core objective of helping clients to ground their
attention in the present to cultivate a mental refuge. The term *mental refuge*
refers to the development of a safe spiritual space by becoming absorbed into
an object of meditation through one of the six senses (focusing attention on
sight, sound, smell, hearing, touch, or mental activities). Through the guidance
of a Buddhist chaplain or other caregiver, clients learn to develop clarity and
stability of mind through various Buddhist mindfulness techniques to foster
a mental refuge. Depending on the client's medical condition, he or she can
develop regular meditative practices throughout the treatment process, such as
mindful breathing, visualization of a safe haven, or sustaining attention of a
particular body part to see the arising and ceasing of sensations. For clients with
stronger muscle tone and eye-hand coordination, mindful tea drinking, callig-
raphy, painting, or other artistic activities are also possible. For clients with

faith in Buddhism, chanting the name of Avalokiteshvara or Amitābha, listening to chanting, reciting mantras, or reading Buddhist scriptures can be useful techniques to help clients foster a mental refuge and soothe their overwhelming emotions. Regardless of choice, the goal is to sustain one's mental attention into the mental refuge to self-soothe from disturbing feelings and thoughts while remaining in equanimity.

To illustrate this model, I will use a hypothetical case example: Mary is a fifty-nine-year-old Chinese female who has thyroid cancer, and she resides in a palliative unit. She appears to be frustrated, lost, and lonely since her admission to palliative care. She also reported many physical problems, such as constipation, fatigue, pain, insomnia, problems with memory, and difficulties with breathing and eating. When the chaplain visited her in the ward, Mary was happy to have someone to talk to, as she felt bored and lonely staying in bed every day. In their first meeting, the chaplain patiently and attentively listened to her and tried to understand her pain and frustration. Mary shared that she used to be an accountant and that she is married, with a daughter who got married two years ago.

With Mary's permission, the chaplain showed Mary different breathing methods, such as intentionally breathing more slowly and deeply, observing her breaths without interference, and focusing on pleasant feelings during her in-breath and out-breath. Mary gradually learned to attend to her breath to soothe her frustrations and tries to breathe mindfully daily. The care provider also worked with Mary to find out her favorite music when she was young and helped Mary to find the music on YouTube, which became another mental refuge to help Mary ground her mind.

Know

The Know phase of treatment is parallel to the concept of wisdom in Buddhism. It helps clients to gain more in-depth knowledge of their suffering through an exploration of their clinging. This phase is an essential step in understanding and ascribing meaning to suffering. In a state of intense grief and loss of hope, many cancer patients tend to reminisce about their lives, resulting in conclusions and self-judgments. Some patients may be proud of their achievements or families, while others have regrets, worries, or unfulfilled wishes. One task for the Buddhist chaplain is to attentively listen to and understand their story of life and help them sort out meanings and themes. Some Buddhist chaplains may suggest journaling, expressive art, or narration to help clients plot a complete story of their lives. For example, Buddhist chaplains can listen to the patient's stories about their life and write it into a story to share with the client, help the client draw out major life events to reflect what the Buddhist chaplain sees the client's meaning of life to be, or let them select favorite songs or lyrics relevant to their lives.

In Mary's example, the Buddhist chaplain tried to raise knowledge on a previous sense of meaning she found in life and to see unnoticed meanings. Mary's primary cause of suffering seems to be her clinging to unfulfilled love from her parents:

MARY: I have done so much for my parents, but how come they only care about my brother?

CHAPLAIN: I see the frustration and resentment on your face. It sounds like genuine love and acceptance from your parents is what you have been yearning for in all these years, but no matter how hard you have tried, you have not felt it.

MARY: I feel like I have wasted my whole life trying to please them . . . and yet, they can only see my brother. I don't know what I have lived for!

CHAPLAIN: Even if your relationship with your parents has not gone the way you wanted, does it really make your life meaningless? Are there other times that you've found meaning?

MARY: I don't know . . . I can at least say I have a great daughter.

Choose

The third phase is *Choose*, which involves making mental and behavioral decisions to choose new volitional activities. The Choose phase focuses on applying the insights that result in daily encounters and fostering the skills needed to make alternative decisions. For some patients, it may have come to the last stage of life, but the mind can still make deliberative choices that result in less suffering. One important strategy to use the deliberative choice to cultivate a healthy state of mind is the recollection of pleasant memories. This technique requires care providers to guide the client to recollect pleasant experiences, especially acts of compassion toward others, and to sustain and expand such mental experiences. With Mary, for example, the Buddhist chaplain tried to help Mary shift from a depressing state of mind to a compassionate one:

CHAPLAIN: What is the best thing you have ever done in life?

MARY: Giving birth to my daughter. She is a very kind girl. She is smart, and she really cares a lot for me.

CHAPLAIN: What is your most precious memory with her?

MARY: I still remember the first time I heard her voice. It was in the operating room. I had been so worried about her throughout the pregnancy, and hearing her cry was such a big relief! I cried. It was a joy. When I got to hold her and look into her cute face, I was so glad that I made the decision to be a mom.

CHAPLAIN: Do you realize your smile while talking about her? It's full of joy and compassion.

MARY: Yes, I can't believe it's thirty-two years ago. . . . Somehow thinking about it makes me feel a lot better.

CHAPLAIN: Yes, I am glad these pleasant memories make you feel better. Coming back to your question, it sounds like you don't feel your parents put enough into their relationship with you, yet you have poured your heart into the relationship with your daughter. From what I have learned, you are a good wife, a respected accountant, and a compassionate mother who has raised a great child. I hope you can remind yourself about all these achievements in life too.

MARY: Thank you . . . I will remember this!

Conclusion

Providing spiritual care for patients with advanced cancer is a difficult task. It may trigger our fear of sickness and death, entitle us to the overwhelming emotions expressed by patients, or elicit our egoistic need to feel that we are helpful to patients. It is vital for care providers to check in with themselves continually to ensure their own psychological well-being. The Note, Know, Choose model can serve as a reference to guide the care provider's approach and techniques. It is important to note that chaplains or others who use this can take any of the ideas and skills to supplement their practice creatively and flexibly with the following considerations.

First and foremost, although the Note, Know, Choose model is a Buddhist teaching-based intervention, good Buddhist chaplains or others who use it should refrain from imposing their religious values and biases on their clients while valuing clients' spirituality and religious beliefs. Every person has an idiosyncratic definition of his or her own faith. Even when the Buddhist chaplain and client both identify themselves as Buddhists, it does not necessarily mean a shared understanding of Buddhist teaching and practice among the two. It is crucial to see each client as a unique individual and humbly learn from their views and see their perspectives during the process of spiritual care. It is also highly important for care providers to follow ethical guidelines of their site of practice as well as their board of certification or registration in order to ensure a professional and nonharming spiritual care relationship.

Second, the Note, Know, Choose model may be applicable to clients suffering from other illnesses, maladies, or critical conditions. Guided by the doctrine of dependent coarising, that every phenomenon is a product of multiple causes and conditions, Buddhist chaplains should learn about the specific physical conditions, mental health conditions, psychological needs, and environmental factors of the client under their care in order to design the optimal course of treatment. In other words, Note, Know, Choose or any other treatment model is nothing more than a tool, and no single tool can fix every problem. A good care provider should always use an open, flexible, and creative mindset in noting the specific conditions contributing to the client's suffering, knowing unskillful habits and mental qualities in the individual, and choosing appropriate techniques to alleviate suffering.

Last but not least, any Buddhist approach begins with cultivation of the care provider. As a practitioner, I believe we should be the first one to benefit from Dhamma and utilize this embodied understanding to benefit others. Just as we prefer a personal trainer stronger than ourselves, we would also prefer a

Buddhist chaplain happier than we are. For this reason, I hope every Buddhist care provider or others who might be inspired by this method can see themselves as one's client and compassionately and wholeheartedly provide care for oneself. We start this committed healing process right at this moment.

13

ACCOMPANYING THE DYING

Applying Noninvasive Dharma for Non-Buddhists

Dian (Dee) Sutawijaya

The Anāthapiṇḍika Sutra tells the story of how the Buddha's disciples, Sāriputta and Ānanda went to visit the wealthy patron Anāthapiṇḍika on his deathbed. Sāriputta sits down by Anāthapiṇḍika's bedside and asks about his level of pain and whether it's increasing or decreasing. Anāthapiṇḍika reports that his pain is intense and increasing. Ānanda then recommends that he keep his mind focused on the Triple Gem (Buddha, Dharma, and Sangha) and relinquish as much of his cravings as he possibly can in his final days. The sutra shows an example of how Buddhist monks cared for the laypeople who were dying. Though the story is very specifically Buddhist, there are elements within it that may be applicable to caring for anyone, no matter their religious background. Pain is often intense at the end of life, and it can be helpful to first take someone's mind off of the pain, onto something more pleasant. Then they can more easily let go of their concerns and find some relaxation and peace in their final days and moments.

I am currently a medical technician at a nursing home in Michigan. But I still return almost annually to my hometown in Indonesia, where I first began learning to adapt my Buddhist views and practices to help people of other faiths. All my family on my father's side are conservative Christians, including my grandmother, whom I was always very close to. We always had fun and joked with each other. My grandma took care of people dying from cancer and was the first person to teach me about end-of-life care. I went home to Indonesia to take care of my grandma when she was dying, because I knew more about the process than anyone else in my family. They were very weary, however, of me trying to convert grandma to Buddhism before she passed on, even standing outside the door to ensure I wasn't proselytizing. But I care for Christians all the time as part of my job and my biggest goal, even as a Buddhist, is simply to allow others to pass away in as peaceful a state as possible.

Most words I say at a patient's bedside are actually from Buddhist teachings, but my grandma is a Christian like them, so I say them in Christian ways. I led her through some breathing practices, but said, "Keep Jesus in your heart." I know she treasured her rosary, so I encouraged her to hold onto it while praying with me: "Dear Jesus, I am thankful for what I have now in this moment. I am blessed. I am grateful for my children who take care of me." It comes from my ideas and practices of gratitude in Buddhism. Yet, I use the words of her tradition, so there was no rejection from her or the rest of my family. I guided her in saying, "May I be happy, Jesus. May I be free from suffering. May I have less pain. May I have peace in my life." Because I know she often worried about her children, I added lines for her to think positively about them too. "May my children also be happy. May my children be free from suffering. May my children find their peace." And then I smiled and asked her jovially, "How about me, your granddaughter? I need your prayers too. Have you prayed for me? I need your blessings too!" She relaxed much more when talking to her and praying with her like this. "Enjoy your present moment. Feel your breath flowing in and out. Feel the air in your lungs." Thus, I guided her through a few minutes of Buddhist meditation, just without the Buddhist terminology.

Of course there are differences between taking care of family and taking care of others for your job, but many of the basic principles are essentially the same. People are naturally afraid of dying. It is important to help them to realize that they are dying, but without scaring them in the process. Before I worked in a nursing home, I was personally very afraid of death. After seeing a dead body, I couldn't sleep for three days. So I understand those worries. Yet, as the Buddha teaches, all of us will age and die. There is no escape. It will show on our bodies. But I try to focus the patients' attention on their life story. Back in Indonesia, I read a Buddhist book that said remembering good deeds the day before death helps you to have a good rebirth when death comes. And of course, from the psychological side, this also helps to relax the mind. I aid people in reflecting on such positive memories. What did they do when they were young? Do they have kids? What are their children doing now? I try to bring those good memories back. I praise all their life accomplishments, no matter how big or small. "Oh, so many successes throughout your life. What a fulfilling life!" Passing away in a nursing home is not fun. Many pass away by themselves, and I never hear anyone say they want to die by themselves. If you can even hold their hand, it makes them feel so much more comfortable.

Try not to deny dying patients their simple joys in life—and help them find those little sparks of joy whenever possible. Sometimes it can require close observation and careful inquiry to find that happiness for them. During the last months of my patient Abigail's life, I noticed she had numerous particularities. She always slept with her radio directly to the right of her head. She previously always slept with a stuffed dog; yet she gave it to her daughter, Becca, since she was dying. I talked with Becca, and it wasn't going to be used so much elsewhere anyway, so Becca brought it back to the nursing home. Both Becca and I were surprised at the difference it made. Abigail smiled so brightly as she went to sleep snuggling that little dog.

We know dying people are often in incredible pain. But I tell them that I hope their pain is subsiding and not increasing. Deep down, there are sometimes moral and ethical struggles I deal with in my profession. We already give patients the best medication we are allowed to give to ease their pain, but sometimes family wants to increase the dosage. I know an increase in dosage leads to quicker death, so even if the family asks for it and receives approval from the medical team, that is not something I take lightly. As a medical technician, I personally administer the morphine. When we up the dosage of morphine to every two hours, people will die within two days. It is my job, and I know that I am not a murderer, but there can be conflicted feelings and sorrow as I administer the medicine.

During such times, I usually take a few minutes to sit by myself and practice *mettā* (loving-kindness) meditation. I send my mettā to them and wish them happiness. After that, I talk to myself and remind myself that this is part of my job and that my intention is to help them decrease their pain. After that, I finally administer the morphine. On those days, I make sure to continue self-care after my shift ends. I walk to the parking lot and sit in my car where I have space to myself. I try to relax as deeply as possible and return my feelings to a more neutral state by listening to music, meditating, or talking to friends over the phone, depending on what feels right that day. My philosophy is, "The inside fire is not to be taken outside; the outside fire is not to be brought inside."

There can be deeply painful added stress for those residents in transition to dementia. They suddenly realize they do not know what they are doing or where they are going. Such residents complain mournfully to me: "I feel stupid. I don't even know what I'm doing." Sometimes they don't realize they are trying to wear shoes on the wrong feet. Realizing your basic mental functions are decreasing can put the mind in further crisis. Their stress is palpable. I try to help them relax in what ways I can. I play music for them, tell them to relax, and enjoy my company. "I know you are tired, but after this, I'll give you some ice cream." Or I give them their favorite tea or something else I know they really enjoy. "Take a deep breath. Relax and enjoy your time. Don't forget to smile!" If I can, I stay with them until they relax and fall asleep. They may even smile while closing their eyes and falling asleep. Just compassionately being with them can make quite a difference during those times.

The stress may increase as dementia progresses. They cry because they don't know things. They wander around and wonder where family members are. My patient Julie didn't remember that her husband passed away. Finding out he passed away years ago was like reliving the grief of that time. As she cried, I calmly remind her, "Let's sit down. Take a deep breath. Remember all the love and laughter you shared with him. Do you feel blessed you lived with his love?" "Yes." "Do you know he loved you too?" "Yes." "Good, good, those are all blessings," I try to warmly tell her while holding her hand. Then we breathe in silence together.

It can be useful to use nicknames and special things that trigger their memory. For example, one patient, Karen, knew we shared the same birthday in December and that everyone called me "Dee." So I always used to smile and say "Dee for December" when I came into her room. By identifying myself like that, she would laugh, smile, and remember who I was. Especially for those with dementia, those tools are very helpful. It can take patience and experimentation. But any way you can identify yourself with certain cues repetitively when introducing yourself each time, you may hit upon the trigger that helps.

A few days before her birthday one year, she entered her dying stages. She mostly slept and didn't respond to anyone. On her birthday, I came to her room to find her son and granddaughter reading the birthday card wishes from her family. She was asleep and not responding to them. I held her hand and said, "Karen, this is 'Dee for December.' I brought a chocolate cake as you requested days ago so we can celebrate our birthday together. Would you open your eyes to see how it looks?" To everyone's surprise, she opened her eyes. We were able to laugh, sing songs, and take pictures together.

The next day, however, I received a report from other staff that she was hitting and punching everybody who tried to touch or care for her. I went to her room, and her son was in there as well. I held Karen's hand and she tried to hit me. I noticed others, including my late grandma, who were in their final days lose control of their reflexes in the same way. Because their organs, nervous system, and other physical functions begin to shut down, they can lose control of their own body. I held her hand and said, "Karen, this is Dee for December." I gently rubbed her hand. "I know you don't mean to hit me. I know how much you love me. I understand this is not an easy stage for you. Some of your bodily functions have started to shut down. It's OK. I'm with you. Take a deep breath. Breathe in. Breathe out. This body is impermanent, but that's natural. Just breathe with me in and out. I sincerely hope the pain is descending."

I usually guide dying residents in that way until they calm down. "Karen, I have to go home, and tomorrow is my day off. If we still have time, I will meet you the day after tomorrow. I pray for your peace and happiness." Unexpectedly, Karen shook my hand gently, and tried to slightly open her eyes. Her voice was so weak, yet she managed to say, "Dee, I love you." In the shock of the moment, her son and I both burst into tears. Beautiful tears of the moment. Her son said, "Mom, this is Dan. I love you, Mom." "I love you, Dan." It was her final sentence—a truly indelible memory. Karen passed away early the next day.

There are some people who think that if people cease responding during their final stages, we are doing little more than waiting for their last breath. But this is completely wrong; their minds are still present. As much as possible, it is important to give all people proper respect in their last moments. It's said that the last sense people have before passing away is their sense of hearing. Even if they do not respond in other ways, they may hear the soothing sound of your voice, your chanting, or your prayers. Even if someone is unconscious, even if someone is under morphine, they still communicate in minor ways. I tell them that I am present for them. I tell them the things I know about them, remind them of the things they like and enjoy. I still talk to them like they are in a regular condition. But they also respond in their own subtle ways.

One day, while taking care of Janice, we were short on staff. It can be challenging to take care of the dying without sufficient staff. In some aspects of care, we really need two people, but we don't have two staff on hand. When a person is dying, it is far more difficult to do simple acts like changing their clothes. We have to do it very gently. Luckily, shortly before Janice passed, we had a second staff person able to help change her clothes. She no longer had the capacity to talk or move, but this does not mean she lost all sense of consciousness. I told Janice, "My friend is over there on the other side of you. We want to turn you onto your side—can you help?" And they do. Even if it's subtle, they help us. I try to respond sincerely from my heart. "Thank you for the opportunity to take care of you. I wish you peace and happiness."

I knew she was going to pass away that night. When people are at that stage, we can tell that it's time. I said, "Enjoy your present moment. Enjoy what you've done through your life. We are here for you, and it is a blessing to take care of you." She couldn't express herself with words, but I was holding her hand as I said these words and felt a small squeeze in response. "I know you are here. Thank you. Thank you for saying hello to me." Those are precious moments; subtle yet beautiful moments when you feel deep down how your effort in their last moments matters to them.

14

IN THE CHARNEL GROUND OF A DYING LATINX MAN

Practicing with Emilio, El Niño Fidencio, and La Santa Muerte

Lourdes Argüelles (Lopon Dorje Khandro), PhD, LMFT

Many years ago, during one long sojourn in India, at the suggestion of a friend who was a *ngakpa* (Tibetan Buddhist nonmonastic tantric practitioner), I rather hesitantly began practicing in a traditional Indian charnel ground. For several days and nights, I kept the company of decaying bodies, feces, blood, and bones, as well as of *sadhus* (Hindu religious ascetics), the occasional Chöd-pa (Tibetan Buddhist Chöd practitioners), stray dogs and monkeys, and a handful of Tibetan Buddhist and Bön (indigenous spiritual tradition of Tibet) practitioners, some of whom regaled me with little boxes of *chulen* (essence pills made by Tibetan doctors and lamas that are designed to replace food and replenish energy), and stale *momos* (Tibetan dumplings). There were also countless beggars who would routinely approach me to ask for coins and food.[1]

During most of my time in the charnel ground I felt apprehensive and shaken to the core of my being, leery of eating any offered food or taking pills, and even refusing assistance to walk through groups of dead bodies without falling. I found myself wanting to discard my Dharma paraphernalia, take a long hot shower at a nice hotel, and run to the closest airport to fly back home. At other times I attempted to distract myself by trying to identify some possible karmic effects that could have propelled me to willingly participate in such a wild scenario and, almost without thinking, to settle into the filthy and scary space that I was now inhabiting. Yet amidst all my fears, mind plays, and plethora of physical discomforts that made it almost impossible for me to focus on my formal Dharma practice, I had the strange sense that I was being prepared for a different type of life than the one I had previously been living back home.

Eventually I had to leave India and return home to attend to an urgent family matter. Once back in the United States, I immediately returned to the everyday life that I had left behind. I sat at least weekly for practice at a beautiful local Dharma center, met often with a kind lama who for years had guided my practice, went back to teaching at the university, and on a monthly basis dutifully crossed the border to briefly help with asylum claims in the trauma-ridden migrant world of the U.S.-Mexico border. Strangely, as time went by and I began spending a bit more time in the border towns of Tijuana and Ciudad Juárez helping to prepare asylum and other immigration claims, I also began missing my Indian charnel ground and reflecting on all the possible lessons I could have better learned there, had it not been for the obstacles of my fears and discomfort.

My kind lama would smile patiently when I talked about yearning to return to my Indian charnel ground practice. Sometimes he would respond by saying, "Not good." At other times he would say, "A charnel ground is any place where you find suffering. So dedicate your Dharma practice to the beings that live in the charnel grounds you are inhabiting in the present moment, including your own internal one."

A few months after my return from India during an evening at a small café in the Mexican border town of Ciudad Juárez, I met Mercedes, a woman who was waiting tables. She told me she had tried to cross the border several times without success and was going to try again the following week. It was the last evening I was to spend in Mexico before returning to my academic post in California. When I told her this, she asked me if I could mail a small box to her son who resided in San Diego at a *casa de curación* (house of healing). She said he was very sick and she wanted to send him an *estampita* (small image) of El Niño Fidencio (a Mexican miracle healer, 1898–1938) and some *remedios caseros* (home remedies).[2] She was afraid that if she mailed the box in Juárez it would get stolen. Against my better judgment, I agreed to mail the box on the other side of the border, but I warned Mercedes that if my car was searched upon crossing the border, U.S. Customs officials would probably think that the remedios were illegal drugs, and I would get in trouble, and the box would be confiscated. Nevertheless, Mercedes begged me to take the box and gave me a big hug and a kiss while saying a prayer to protect me from harm. She then assured me repeatedly that El Niño Fidencio would look after me.

The following day I crossed the border with the estampita and remedios box in my backpack and without any trouble. I had planned that once I was in San Diego, I would FedEx the box to Mercedes's son, but when I read the address, I realized that on my way home I would be passing by the facility where he was living. I decided then to deliver the box in person.

The door of the small house where the box was addressed was open, and when I walked in, the three men who were sitting in the living room watching TV at first paid little attention to me. To one side of the TV set was an altar with pictures that I assumed were from family members and also pictures of Catholic saints. In front of the pictures there were several small glasses of water, a bottle of rum, cigars, and freshly cut flowers. One of the men, who said his name was Gonzalo, welcomed me when I told him that I had come to deliver a box to Emilio. He immediately noticed my interest in the altar and said that he was the *cuidador* (caretaker) and that the pictures were of his and his wife's ancestors and ancestors of the men that were currently living with them. He added, "The others are from *la virgen* [the Virgin of Guadalupe, Catholic patron saint of Mexico] and saints." Then he asked, "Do you know their names?" "Yes, I think so," I responded, as I tried to remember the pictures from the altars of the Catholic churches that I had frequented as a child in my native country. I proceeded to list la Virgen de Guadalupe, San Judas, San Cipriano, San Diego, and San Santiago. Then I looked to the small table tucked away in a corner and saw a stand-alone picture of an amber-colored skeletal female figure dressed as a bride, holding a scythe, and surrounded by candles, dried flowers, dollar bills, bones, and other offerings. Gonzalo smiled and said, "I imagine you do not know Nuestra Señora de la Santa Muerte (Our Lady of the Holy Death)." "Yes, actually I do," I responded, feeling somewhat proud. Gonzalo nodded and smiled again. Then he said, "She is the *patrona* (patron) of this house." Shortly thereafter, Mercedes's son, Emilio, came into the room assisted by a woman whom Gonzalo introduced as his wife and said she was a *curandera* (traditional healer). Gonzalo's wife's name was Azucena, and she invited me to sit down.

Emilio was a tall, frail young man who had some difficulty walking and had many Kaposi's sarcoma lesions visible on his arms and on part of his face. He seemed to be in his twenties. After I handed the box to Emilio, Gonzalo asked the other men to help him in the garden, and to leave Emilio, Azucena, and me alone for a while.

Emilio opened the box, and he seemed elated when he saw the contents. He took out the picture of El Niño Fidencio, which came in its own little frame, and put the bag of remedios in his pocket. Azucena put the box away in the drawer of an old desk, on top of which there were even more pictures of Catholic saints and more glasses of water, along with freshly cut flowers, a few cans of beer, and several candles of different colors.

Emilio stayed leaning quietly near the main altar after he carefully placed the picture of El Niño Fidencio next to San Diego. Azucena, however, began talking nonstop and asking me all sorts of questions. Before I had a chance to respond to any of her questions, she said, "This is a casa de curación and I am a curandera. The men that are here have AIDS. I am telling you this," she continued, "because I can tell you can be trusted." She paused, and when I did not respond, she continued, "I will tell you some other time why you are here." I felt she was trying to elicit some reaction from me, but what reaction she anticipated I could not guess. Suddenly I was aware of a feeling of wanting to leave and go home, somewhat akin to the feeling I had when I wanted desperately to leave the Indian charnel ground. However, not only did I end up staying at the casa de curación for several hours that day, I returned many more times during the span of almost a year.

"You are meant to be here," Azucena said repeatedly. "It is not a coincidence," she added. "I will tell you more another day." She then proceeded to tell me more about her casa de curación, which she said was also a *casa de oración* (prayer house).

The casa de curación was a group home where six men from Mexico and Central America with full-blown AIDS and other illnesses lived with Gonzalo and Azucena, who were both trained certified nursing assistants. The home was supported by governmental monies and by donations from an NGO. The nearby medical center provided medical treatment and follow-up for the men, though Gonzalo confided that the allopathic treatments were supplemented

at la casa de curación by many potions and Mexican-style foods and comple-
mented by the necessary prayers, *limpias* (cleansings), and rituals.

Before coming to the United States from Mexico, Azucena had been trained
as a curandera by her grandmother. Gonzalo had studied with several healers in
Mexico to become a *yerbero* (traditional herbalist). A *sobador* (traditional masseuse) that they had both known in Mexico visited the casa de curación quite
often and treated the residents as well as Gonzalo and Azucena. Native herbs
were grown in the casa's garden and also purchased from a nearby *botánica* (traditional botanical store) where incense, oils, herbs, candles, and other ritual
items were also obtained. Azucena, who unlike Gonzalo was documented,
would occasionally cross the U.S.-Mexico border at Tijuana and proceed to
Ensenada, where she could obtain certain remedios unavailable in the United
States.

At the request of Azucena, and with Emilio's consent, I began to visit the
casa de curación once a week. I usually stayed for a couple of hours, and I got to
know Emilio well. We talked about his AIDS diagnosis two years before, his
diabetes, and his severe kidney problems. He confided that he knew that he was
going to die soon and was preparing for his death. Azucena did not try to dissuade him from thinking about an early death and encouraged him to prepare
for it. She asked him to invoke La Santa Muerte more frequently. Sometimes
she would look at me and say, "You can help him." I would protest and say that
I knew little about how to help Emilio and even less about La Santa Muerte.
Though I did not say it openly, I would often imply that I was not looking forward to learning more about this somewhat controversial skeletal saint whom
I considered a worldly deity not worth invoking, a deity that was increasingly
being associated with drug users and cartels. Emilio repeatedly tried to dissuade
me from thinking negatively about his patrona. He would say that La Santa
Muerte was nonjudgmental and tried to help everyone, whether saints or sin-
ners, without preference. For Emilio and for Azucena, her supreme neutrality
had to do with the fact that Death treats everyone equally.

A few weeks later, Mercedes, Emilio's mother, crossed into the United
States, made it to San Diego, and moved nearby. She and Azucena often joined
my conversations with Emilio. Then, Emilio and I gradually began to meet
separately from them to discuss religion, La Santa Muerte, El Niño Fidencio,

death, rebirth, and other matters that seemed of interest to one or both of us. A Catholic, Mercedes introduced me to the healing work she was now doing in connection with the Fidencista Christian Church, a Mexican church based on the teachings of El Niño Fidencio to which she now belonged.

Slowly, I began to look forward to my visits to la casa de curación, where, in addition to interesting conversation, I would occasionally get a free *sobada* (traditional Mexican massage). Azucena would often interrupt my conversation with Emilio to serve both of us strong-tasting juices that she said were made with special herbs that we both needed in order to clean our energies. Surprisingly, I would drink these without any fear or apprehension. Emilio would occasionally take me into his room, which he shared with another resident, to show me one of the various books he had on religion, including several on Buddhism. He said that he had become very interested in this topic while at San Diego State University, where he had studied for a year before being diagnosed with AIDS.

Several months went by, and I never missed my weekly visits to la casa de curación. Emilio began to get sicker, and Gonzalo took him to the hospital on an emergency basis a couple times. The day after one of those hospital visits, Emilio asked me if there was a Buddhist practice or ritual that I could do with him or for him. I asked him for what purpose he wanted the practice or ritual and, to my surprise, he did not say he wanted it to help with his health.

"I leave anything having to do with my health to El Niño Fidencio and La Santa Muerte," he said. "Buddhists are supposed to try to help others all the time, and I want to do that," he added. "Why?" I asked. "I think this is why I am in this world, and La Santa Muerte wants us to use all means to help ourselves and others. I can learn a new way from you," he answered.

I first provided Emilio with background information and careful instructions about Tonglen (Giving and Taking Practice), which was my main Dharma practice at the time.[3] A week later, we started practicing some visualizations together. Emilio began by visualizing El Niño Fidencio, who he said was his and his mother's main teacher, above the crown of his head. I visualized H. H. the 14th Dalai Lama above my crown. We then began meditating on great compassion and on how wonderful it would feel if everyone were completely released from suffering and were able to enjoy happiness. Emilio was very pleased. Later he would tell me that during his last visit to the hospital, where he had witnessed quite a lot of suffering in the emergency room, he felt the energy of El Niño Fidencio coming down into his body through his crown. He felt more strongly than ever before, the desire to help all the patients and anyone else in the world who was suffering. Years before this visit to the hospital, one of El Niño Fidencios's *cajitas* (mediums), named Estela, whom Emilio had met in Mexico, had urged that he extend compassion and help for anyone in need, even to his own father, who had been very violent with him, and his mother. For some time he had forgotten this advice, but more recently, after he had become sick, every evening before going to bed he thought about the need for compassion for everyone. While praying to El Niño Fidencio, he would ask El Niño to send good energies to this planet that would heal those sick of both mind and body in the present, past, and future. Emilio told me that, in addition to the living who were suffering in the present, he was concerned about his deceased ancestors who were unable to find peace and were still lurking around him and the rest of his family. He also said he was worried about the children still to be born in a century where great catastrophes and thus great sufferings were being predicted.

Emilio and I began a series of discussions on topics such as ancestors and prophecies. He shared with me various prophecies from his Mesoamerican culture, and I shared with him the Buddhist teachings about the Era of the Five Degenerations.[4] We also shared our concern for beings which he called "restless ancestors" and that I called "beings caught between the *bardos* (in-between states) of death and rebirth." Azucena and Gonzalo, along with one of the men living in la casa, sometimes joined in the discussions. Although we disagreed on some minor points, we agreed on the need for cultivating compassion for all living beings, including animals, to which they added the need to include their beloved plants—which they believed were very much alive and aware. We also talked at length about our own self-cherishing as the main source of our suffering and how Tonglen practice could be very helpful in reducing our tendency to cling to our "I." They related especially to my comments regarding the need to avoid thinking of things as "mine." They all concurred that everything belonged to everybody, and in the end to nobody, as La Santa Muerte had taught them.

By the time Emilio and I began to practice Tonglen a few weeks after our visualization practices and our initial discussions about suffering, compassion, and prophecies, all the members of la casa de curación as well as Mercedes and the sobador were on board. When we began practicing breathing in sufferings in the form of black smoke, Emilio and everyone else except me paused. On everyone's behalf, Emilio asked me if it would be OK if they could imagine some of the suffering coming in the form of smoke of different colors, including white, because suffering came in many colors. They also said they wanted to visualize the light coming out as we exhaled in a variety of colors. The use of many colors to visualize the breath and the light seemed to them like a much better way to do the practice.

Together we all practiced various forms of Tonglen once a week for about two months. We continued to visualize the Dalai Lama and El Niño Fidencio on our crowns, and their pictures were placed on a Tonglen altar that Gonzalo and Azucena constructed in a covered part of their backyard. Every week, through our breath, we sent offerings to all, as we also took in suffering from ourselves, from all types of beings who were living at the time, the restless dead, and the children yet to be born in these times. At the end of the practice sessions, Azucena and Emilio said prayers to La Santa Muerte. They thanked her for encouraging them to think about the well-being of everyone without exception and to keep the awareness that we were all equal because all of us were destined to die.

Emilio's health continued to deteriorate, and he began begging his mother to take him back to Mexico where he said he wanted to die. Mercedes in turn begged him to remain in the United States, hoping that his doctors could arrange a kidney transplant that would extend his life. She also hoped that the treatments he was receiving at the San Diego hospital and at la casa would prolong his life. In the end she relented and began to organize a quick trip back home. Azucena, Gonzalo, and I began to plan a ceremony to say good-bye to Emilio for which Gonzalo hurriedly began to build two more altars to both honor Emilio and those he believed were now Emilio's two most important spiritual patrons as he drew closer to death: La Santa Muerte and Buddha Amitābha, whose Pure Land Emilio seemed to have developed a strong attraction for after he heard me recite the Prayer to be Reborn in Dewachen (Amitābha's Pure Land). Both altars faced west because it is said that La Santa Muerte always reminds her devotees that her true home is in the land of the dead, which is in the west, and because Gonzalo remembered Emilio mentioning that Amitābha was the Buddha of the Western Paradise.

At midnight on a cold evening a week after the feast of the Days of the Dead was celebrated at la casa de curación, we held our ceremony for Emilio. It was attended by more than one hundred people who were relatives and friends of the residents. Some were also devotees of El Niño Fidencio or La Santa Muerte. The ceremony was conducted by Azucena, who appeared to be in a trance, and by my Tibetan lama, who joined us for the occasion. Throughout the night, I assisted Emilio to stand up as well as to kneel at different times during the ceremony. Azucena invoked and prayed to La Santa Muerte on his behalf and my lama recited the Prayer to be Reborn in Dewachen. At the end of the ceremony, Azucena burned incense, the lama bestowed blessings on all seen and unseen beings who were present, and Gonzalo passed around several trays of *plantas sacramentales* (sacramental plants) that the owner of the local botánica had donated. Emilio, who was clutching the picture of El Niño Fidencio that I had brought to him from Juárez, approached the altars and bowed several times. Then he placed dried flowers on La Santa Muerte's altar and fresh flowers on Amitābha's. He hugged me and handed me the box I had brought him. Inside were a picture of El Niño Fidencio, an image of La Santa Muerte, and some remedios.

The following day, Mercedes and Emilio left for Mexico. Not long after, she called me and said that Emilio had just died peacefully. I immediately called my lama and he performed Phowa (a Tibetan Buddhist practice of ejection of consciousness at the time of death), and I began a forty-nine-day ritual for the dead based on the *Bardo Thodol* (aka *The Tibetan Book of the Dead*). I soon called Azucena to let her know about Emilio's passing. She whispered a brief prayer and asked me, "Do you know now why you came to my house?" I told her I did.

I never returned physically to la casa de curación, but I remained in touch with Azucena and Gonzalo for a couple of years until they too returned to Mexico. They said they were moving back to a house they had purchased in the Mexican village where Azucena was born and where they hoped Mercedes and her new husband would join them. Their plan was to devote themselves to helping people better their lives, heal from illness, and become friends with death before their own dying process began. When I last talked to her, Azucena promised that she and Gonzalo would both keep me in their prayers to El Niño Fidencio and especially to La Santa Muerte.

I often return mentally to my Indian charnel ground and to la casa de curación where I began to learn not to seek to escape the inescapable, but to work with whatever presents itself. These have been incredibly valuable lessons that help me to navigate the multiple converging and compounding crises of our present moment.

These experiences also encouraged me a few years ago to move beyond my university and counseling offices to outreach to vulnerable people who, for a multiplicity of political, socioeconomic, and cultural reasons, do not receive care and possibly will never receive care in mainstream institutional settings. Ever since I made that move, I have been privileged to assist mostly, though not exclusively, Latinx men and women who receive their physical, emotional, and spiritual care in community group homes or who are cared for by relatives, neighbors, curanderas, and even strangers in their own homes, in squatter houses, in shelters, in their cars, or in the streets on both sides of the border. In these third or communal spaces, where bonds of affection often take precedence over professionalized help, I now visit and serve as a caring friend, a professional helper, a Dharma practitioner, or simply as an old immigrant who is known to be always on the lookout for boxes of spiritual inspiration and remedios to help replenish her flagging energies.

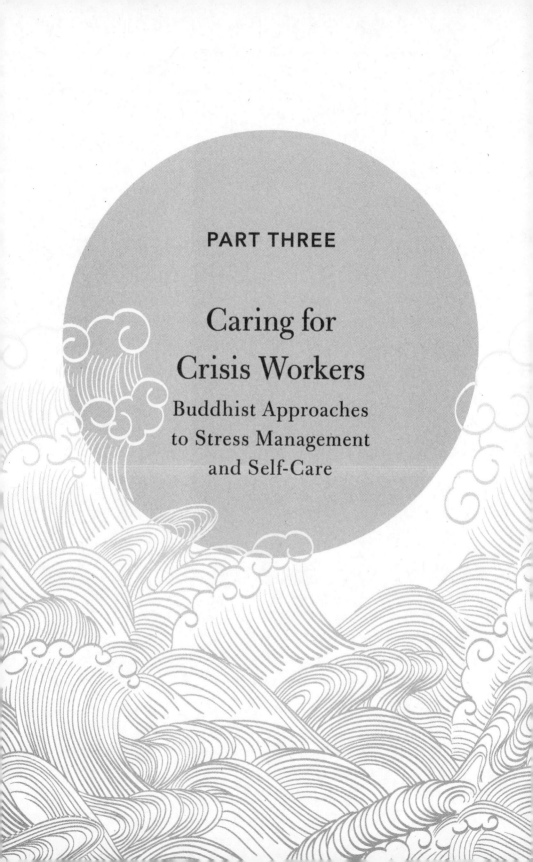

PART THREE

Caring for Crisis Workers

Buddhist Approaches
to Stress Management
and Self-Care

15

REFLECTING CLEAR MOONLIGHT

When Modern Chaplaincy Embodies a Living Koan

Shushin R. A. Peterson

Great Master Ma was feeling unwell. The temple superintendent asked him, "Teacher, how are you these days?" The great master said, "Sun Face Buddha, Moon Face Buddha."

—CASE 3, BLUE CLIFF RECORD (BDK English Tripitaka 75)

Part 1: The Case of Master Ma

I received a call from the Chaplain Services office saying that a patient was in crisis and the nursing staff hoped we would be able to help. Upon entering the darkened room, I saw a thin man rocking back and forth, holding his leg and weeping. Looking up at me he said, "They just told me they have to cut off my leg or else I'll die." I could feel the energy in the room, the desperation and the fear. I could also feel my own anxiety. I had no medical power, no ability to restore a limb to life, but the man's sobs pleaded, demanded, for something to be done.

Spiritual caregivers are often tempted by this siren's call to fix a point of crisis. It persuades us that if we just do the right thing or move fast enough, the crisis will be resolved. It is even more seductive because, for other types of care-givers, the necessity of speedy and decisive action is sometimes true—if doctors act fast enough, the impact of illness and injury can be greatly averted. The same is true for firefighters, police officers, and other first responders. Crisis often demands action, but sitting across from this weeping man, I knew that as a chaplain there was nothing I could do to heal his leg.

Confronted with such acute suffering, spiritual care providers may get hooked by the seduction of solving and fixing. If we can just reach a family member on the phone, then things will be OK. If we can only provide the right holy book, pamphlet, or referral to the social worker, then everything will be fine. Even without crisis, it is easy to get caught by the idea that care is offered through solving problems, providing meal cards, or quoting scripture. Sometimes these actions may be helpful, but their utility exists only as support for a deeper form of spiritual care. By itself, a focus on "fixing" may cause more harm than good. A patient once expressed his anger when, after sharing his helplessness at being unable to afford the transfer of a family member's body from the coroner's office, he was offered a $20 meal card by Chaplain Services. In moments of physical and emotional crisis, in the presence of this compunc-tion to act, how can chaplains respond in a wholesome way?

In Zen Buddhism, koans, or "public cases," are meant to be examined in community. In koan practice, a teacher and student examine these questions, statements, or small anecdotes together and attempt to manifest the deeper teaching embodied in them. Koans can appear nonsensical or as a non sequi-tur, but applied in the context of a deeper spiritual practice, they point toward truths about ourselves, our relationships with others, and the nature of our real-ity. As Chan (Zen) Buddhism developed in Song Dynasty China during the twelfth century, many influential koans were collected into an anthology called the *Blue Cliff Record*. Due to the anthology's popularity, commentaries by later masters were attached to the koans, helping exemplify and expand their under-lying meaning. Applying this wisdom to our modern day, we will first discuss how the third case in the *Blue Cliff Record*, "Master Ma Was Feeling Unwell," can be a direct response to the predicament of all chaplains when feeling the call for action in moments of crisis, as well as an overarching orientation through which to view spiritual care in a medical setting. We will then briefly examine how Master Xuedou's commentary to this case may assist chaplains or others in preparing to provide spiritual care.

The koan begins with the temple superintendent checking in on Master Ma, who is unwell. The superintendent behaves like a chaplain in many ways. Just like a chaplain, the superintendent is a religious professional who has duties beyond a strictly ritual function, including the care of those who are ill. As the case opens, the superintendent, acting as chaplain, immediately falls into the trap of focusing on external solutions by asking about Master Ma's health and comfort. The superintendent is not a doctor, and yet he is hooked by the immediacy of Master Ma's illness and becomes fixated on addressing it. He struggles to understand that chaplains are not called to address physical ailments—especially in today's health-care settings, which already orient around doctors, nurses, and other specialists in physical health.

Our well-being is impacted by our physical health, and also by our mental, emotional, and spiritual health. In Zen Buddhism, we are taught that all beings have the potential to become Buddhas. To manifest this potential, known in Mahāyāna Buddhism as Buddha Nature, is to operate in the world free from the controlling influence of our attachments and assumptions. The more we are able to access this potential, the more we will experience the contentment of a life not fettered by the stresses of clinging to transient pleasures. Our suffering springs from our resistance to the stresses and unpleasant aspects of life, reinforced by our insistence that reality conform to our expectations. If our suffering arises from our assumptions and desires, then the tranquility of Buddhahood can be considered our natural or original state, before the friction of our attachments clouded our world. Far more can be said about the actual status of Buddha Nature and how it relates to other core Buddhist teachings, but our work as spiritual care providers is rarely to explain teachings. Rather it is to embody them through relationship, as Master Ma will show us. Our intrinsic wholeness and potential for liberation may become deemphasized when ill, and even more obscured in crisis situations as we are pulled away from ourselves by devastating events, illnesses, and loss.

Chaplains are asked to engage with patients during some of the most desperate points in their lives. Even outside a specific point of crisis, patients may already be disadvantaged in a health-care setting. Numerous patients have described to me how they feel like they lose their identity when they come to the hospital. Their clothing is taken from them, and they are referred to by numbers, room, or diagnosis. Especially in situations where infection control is a paramount concern, patients are barred from having friends and family visit, and the people who can interact with them are gowned, gloved, and masked, further obstructing human connection. During pandemics, natural disasters, or other catastrophes, medical staff are pushed to their own limits, overworked and carrying their own burdens, which may then be perceived as arrogance or disregard by their patients, all of which further enforces feelings of dehumanization and disconnection. A common theme I have observed among Vietnam War–era veterans at our hospital is that they transfer their experiences of social rejection upon returning from overseas in the 1970s onto their current understanding of why their medications are late or their meals are cold. Uprooted from their homes, surrounded by strangers, most of what normally reinforces a person's identity and security is removed. This lack of personal grounding makes the patient all the more vulnerable to the fear, loss, and grief that may arrive at any time: sudden news of amputation, cancer, stroke, a future walled in by a serious diagnosis, or any other aspect of the suffering contained in old age, sickness, and death.

In this darkness, chaplains may bring hope and comfort. The greatest hope found in Mahāyāna Buddhist teachings is the knowledge that our original Buddha Nature is complete, pure, and unchanging. Our Buddha Nature is neither increased nor decreased by external conditions, and it cannot be degraded, broken, or lost due to outside circumstances. Our intrinsic nature cannot be damaged, but it can be forgotten, especially when we are drawn outside ourselves due to an emergency or simple everyday distraction. The greatest service a chaplain can offer is accompanying our patients back to touch that original source of wholeness that forms the foundation of our mutual interconnection with each other. Master Ma understood all of this and hoped to join in a more sincere form of therapeutic relationship with the superintendent—as well as with current chaplains floundering with superficial conversations about hospital food or wait times—when he said:

Sun Face Buddha, Moon Face Buddha.

Master Ma, skillfully flipping the relationship and becoming the chaplain for the superintendent, avoided the pitfall of "fixing" the superintendent's superficial viewpoint by lecturing him about proper behavior. Rather, Master Ma entered into a mutual relationship with the superintendent that upholds the potential they both have to manifest awakening. Through this new relationship, Master Ma demonstrates that the greatest service we can offer others is when we understand and intentionally mirror back their inherent wholeness. When we hold our patients as complete despite their challenges, a safe and spiritually quiet space is created for our patients to find grounding and reconnect with themselves, just as the moon is able to shine by mirroring the light of the sun.

By connecting and existing with our patients in the moment of their suffering, rather than interacting with them as if their medical condition, emotional turmoil, or point of crisis embodies their entirety, there is an opportunity for both the chaplain and the patient to exist in mutuality with each other. One patient who was in strict isolation due to COVID-19 received word that his son, whom he had last seen and argued with, was killed in a car accident and the patient would be unable to leave the hospital to attend the funeral. Trapped inside the hospital, he was tearing himself apart. Through validating his emotional reactions, rather than trying to get him to calm down, and exploring his understandings of fatherhood and responsibility that shaped his grief, we were able to sit in his suffering until the sharpest forms of his pain had run their course. He then felt able to reach out to his family and begin the process of grief, meaning-making, and healing. When patients are able to reorient back toward themselves and touch the understanding that they are already enough, they are able to better face their current crisis. This grounded remembering then allows them to navigate a proactive course toward a more meaningful, spiritually healthy response.

A key spiritual practice in Zen Buddhism is exploring the union of the absolute and the relative. In the same way, truly seeing our patients requires the parallel process of being able to hold them as whole and complete as they are, while simultaneously acknowledging and working with the emotional distress, interpersonal relationship issues, or medical challenges they might be facing. While the superintendent was hooked by Master Ma's external illness, there is an equally dangerous pitfall at the opposite end of the spectrum in overly simplistic optimism. Whether a caregiver offers such superficial optimism due to overconfidence or as a way to avoid feelings of distress or helplessness, disregarding the full situation a patient faces ignores a fundamental part of who the patient is at this moment.

When the moon shines, it reflects back the light of the sun—but to a much smaller degree. Unlike the sun, this reduced intensity allows the moon to be directly seen. Depending on how a chaplain chooses to understand this orientation, we might either be the moon or the sun. As the moon, we gently mirror back a patient's distress in such a way that it is no longer scorching, allowing the patient to directly engage with it. As the sun, we are gently illuminating a whole and complete human being who had been covered by the darkness of their suffering. Chaplains and patients flow between both perspectives throughout the encounter, occasionally exploring, occasionally validating, and upholding both orientations at the same time within their relationship. Through these orientations, by examining the patient's situation together with the chaplain, the relationship allows the patient to rediscover and better understand that they already possess all the emotional and spiritual resources needed to move forward.

I once worked with a patient suffering from both skin and mouth cancer, resulting in a decaying pit where most of his right cheek and eye had been. The patient refused my visits several times due to his deformity. However, through holding the truth that he, just as much as anyone, was still spiritually whole, and reaching out to the patient with that understanding, he eventually allowed a visit. It resulted in us being able to develop a longer relationship where we processed his desire for discharge and home hospice care, and to explore both the joy he still had from being in nature as well as the pain of social isolation and deformity. Ultimately, he also reflected on his views of death and how to create what he viewed as a good death for himself. It is difficult to think how he would have responded to a relationship centered solely on his disease or, conversely, a caregiving approach that disregarded it entirely.

Part of this rediscovery of agency and wholeness may involve chaplains responding to limited physical or practical needs, such as getting an extra blanket or checking to see when medications will arrive. This allows patients to see their own worth reflected in the chaplain's willingness to help. However, when addressing physical needs, it is good to remain sensitive to the deeper causes of spiritual distress and not follow the superintendent's example of focusing on purely external aspects of the patient's situation. Much greater comfort can come from sincere presence and willingness to journey with someone in their suffering.

Offering such a sincere presence requires developing the skill and discernment to sit within moments of suffering without being drawn toward the need to fix or resolve the situation. Formal koan practice usually encourages nonconceptual, nonrational realization of truths, which come from holding the koan over a long period of time. In the same way, developing the ability to be with others in their suffering is less a matter of formal academic instruction and more about holding the question of how best to be in relationship with our patients. Attending classes and workshops about active listening or cultural sensitivity can be useful in strengthening practical skills, but such skills must be backed by a deeper spiritual orientation that, like much of Buddhist practice, is easy to conceptualize but requires effort and experience in relationship to embody. Master Xuedou, who commented on Master Ma's koan, seemed well aware of both the difficulty and necessity in being spiritually grounded enough to do this work. In his commentary on the koan, we see a path laid out to prepare ourselves to be with others in their suffering, a journey which, for many of us, may require great courage.

Part 2: The Commentary of Master Xuedou

Sun-faced Buddha, moon-faced Buddha; what kind of people were the ancient emperors? For twenty years I have struggled; how many times have I gone down into the blue dragon's cave for you! This distress is worth recounting; clear-eyed Chan practitioners should not take it lightly.

—MASTER XUEDOU, Commentary to "Master Ma Was Feeling Unwell"
(BDK English Tripitaka 75)

The process of mirroring someone's intrinsic nature can only take place within a mutual relationship. These relationships, however, might face challenges if a caregiver is not spiritually prepared for this work. Master Xuedou, a Song Dynasty monastic, laid out a process centuries ago that, surprisingly, matches the clinical education and spiritual formation of modern chaplains. Through his commentary on the case of Master Ma, we can see how spiritual care providers may cultivate the personal understanding needed to enter into potentially difficult relationships with others as "Sun Face Buddha, Moon Face Buddha."

A pervasive clinical myth is that spiritual care professionals leave ourselves—our baggage, our assumptions, our myths—at the door when we interact with patients. This view seems present when Anton Boison, the founder of modern chaplaincy, suggested we view others as "living human documents," though in fairness this new lens was an advancement over viewing patients as mechanical objects to be repaired. Many chaplains are now moving away from this implicit view of patients as objects to be analyzed and toward spiritual care that comes through entering into relationship with our patients. We therefore bring all of ourselves, whether we like it or not, into the room with us.

Spiritual care providers are human and we are equally susceptible to being drawn outside ourselves and losing our grounding during times of crisis. As humans, our empathetic nature makes it possible for us to take on other people's burdens as if they were our own or to project our own traumas and anxieties onto those in front of us. A fellow chaplain once spoke with a dying patient who was processing regret and reconciliation with his adult daughter over abuse he had inflicted on her growing up. The chaplain's own child was the same age as the patient's at the time of the abuse, and the revulsion, disgust, and protectiveness rose so sharply in the chaplain that it threatened the therapeutic relationship. In situations like this it is possible for chaplains to experience vicarious suffering just as acute as those we encounter.

To be capable of providing a space where patients can reconnect with their own nature and work toward healing requires a chaplain to have thoroughly delved into their own emotional and spiritual histories. In the commentary, Master Xuedou wonders what type of people are capable of laying this groundwork. Many of our personal histories are marked by acute suffering. We all have varying experiences with broken relationships, trauma, grief, and loss. Often, for us to survive these experiences, we have had to block those memories and avoid them as much as possible. However, these wounds still fester within us even as our surface selves appear whole and healthy. These wounds are the cave of the blue dragon, our deepest wells of shame, fear, anger, and all the emotional and psychological burdens and assumptions that we have accrued during our wanderings in life.

Old wounds, unexplored biases, and preconceptions are often so pervasive within our emotional landscape that we don't recognize when we have slipped into old patterns. Our assumptions appear as truths that we do not even question: "Of course those who are older than me are wiser. How can preserving a patient's life at any cost not be our highest priority? No one ever wants to die unless they are mentally unstable." Dōgen Zenji, founder of Sōtō Zen Buddhism, famously said, "To study Buddhism is to study the self. To study the self is to forget the self." In our fast-paced individualistic society, which already gives us a strong sense of self, Zen Buddhists might be tempted to skip immediately to the end of this process and start with the forgetting. This type of spiritual bypass seems very safe, since it allows us to avoid entering a cave that shows us who we are, stripped of our artificial self-conception. To see ourselves as we truly are is very distressing, as Master Xuedou tells us. Unfortunately, if we do not embark on this journey of discovery, it allows all these buried wounds within ourselves to continue to be actively avoided or quietly ignored while they retain influence over us.

We once pointed out to a chaplain that a female patient was subtly commenting that she felt the chaplain-patient relationship was easing into something deeper and more intimate. The chaplain, having internalized childhood messages of being a social outcast, was unable to see the signs of growing enmeshment and reacted quite strongly when these signals were pointed out. Disbelief that anyone would view him romantically rose within him. Anger also rose as he realized that he might have missed similar cues in the past, and his life of social isolation may have been due to his own myths of personal worthlessness rather than any true deficiency. Defensiveness also flared within him over feeling like he was being accused of intentionally entrapping a patient in a predatory relationship, as well as self-recrimination over not having seen the signs himself or ensuring healthy spiritual care for a patient. To address wounds like these, that are so deep they can define reality for us, and to begin our own healing, we must go down and meet our blue dragons—not once or twice, but time and time again. Only after we are aware and have reconciled our emotions, narratives, and history will we be in a position to help others without our own story hijacking our relationships.

Viewing the journey into the blue dragon's cave as a metaphor for personal exploration is not a new interpretation. Buddhists in many traditions have practiced this type of self-study long before Western psychology embarked on its own exploration of the mind. However, this journey into the cave takes on new relevance when viewed within the therapeutic relationship between patient and spiritual care provider. Board certified chaplains are required to have four units of clinical pastoral education (CPE), which emphasizes patient visits backed by supervised education with a cohort of fellow chaplains (see chapter 23, "The Path to Buddhist Chaplaincy," for more details about this educational process). One major aspect of CPE is the continual work of going "down into the blue dragon's cave" time and again and uncovering our true selves. This is done through CPE's foundational clinical practice of "act, process, act," both at the bedside and later during formal reports of meaningful encounters. In these reports, CPE students examine how they responded to certain patients or conversations, process where these responses came from, and what motivations or assumptions were behind their actions. When encountering similar situations, they then act again, this time informed by what was discovered through processing the previous events.

This core practice is enacted within a framework of didactics, spiritual exploration, and collaboration within a cohort. The cohort mirrors Buddhist understandings of the importance of the Sangha. The distress that such personal exploration can cause requires communal support in a trusted environment to thoroughly process and integrate, and like the enmeshed chaplain above, we all have blind spots that, despite our best intentions and most concerted practice, may go unnoticed without peers equally dedicated to this path of understanding. Both Master Ma and Master Xuedou lived in communities that upheld their cultivation, and many aspects of this communal spiritual support is found in the CPE cohort. In my own cohort we grew together, clashing as our assumptions were challenged, breaking down as we faced realizations about our lives and choices, and building community in order to risk being truly known for who we are underneath our public facade. Going through this process, we felt the weight of our histories and assumptions ease with new self-awareness. The impact of this new understanding can be far-reaching. Our supervisor once shared that half of married CPE educator candidates, who go through more self-discovery training than many chaplains, divorce as they discover and integrate previously hidden subcurrents that influenced their life choices.

By "recounting this distress," chaplains become grounded enough to either be Moon Face Buddhas, reflecting the Sun Face of our patients' intrinsic nature, or Sun Face Buddhas, illuminating deeper understandings and allowing the Moon Face of our patients to shine. This process does not mean that our histories and traumas cease to affect us. By understanding ourselves, we eventually arrive at a space of freedom where we are not compelled to follow the habitual compunction to relive our past traumas with our patients as surrogate antagonists, but to make new choices. The painful examination of past times when I have been manipulated allowed me to understand my disproportionate emotional reaction when our interdisciplinary team discovered that a patient whom I felt I had a deep and trusting relationship with had fabricated many of his complaints. Master Xuedou's process of introspection allowed me to understand why such intense emotions arose within me and gave me the space to proactively decide how to move forward with the patient given this new context, rather than lashing out with the anger and hurt of my previous experiences or simply abandoning the relationship. Through this process, chaplains are, in a sense, "forgetting ourselves," as Dōgen reflected, but this is a new type of forgetting where past traumas no longer control us.

This challenge seems daunting, but we are all capable of this work. Just as our patients are whole and complete despite their challenges, we the spiritual care providers are complete too, despite our challenges. We learn to rely on our own intrinsic wholeness as we continue to meet the suffering of the world. When we courageously venture into the darkness again and again, our dragons cease to be adversaries and slowly become allies whose fierceness can teach us to better empathize and bear witness to similar struggles that our patients face. When I sat with a recently bereaved son, my own experiences of death and loss helped mirror the son's grief, allowing his father's decline, dementia, and death to be unique but not unknown. Having explored our own wholeness in the midst of suffering, spiritual caregivers can more fully uplift aspects of our patients' story that support them or aspects that they might be avoiding. We might even be able to offer a model of how such experiences may be cared for and integrated.

The process of self-discovery is imperative in offering effective spiritual care, especially during times of crisis. For both caregivers and patients, extraordinary circumstances strip us of the pleasant distractions and easy comforts of our everyday lives. In crisis, spiritual caregivers are called to hold the distress of others, while also navigating our own reactions to the same events, which can stretch limited internal resources. If we are unaware when our wounds are activated, we may counter-transfer our own distress onto our patients, allowing the memory of our suffering to be reborn into the reality of this moment and continue the cycle of pain. The deeper we have delved into the blue dragon's cave, the more space we will have cleared out to hold the experiences of others without it overflowing in unhealthy ways. This is why it takes several years to become a Board Certified Chaplain, and moreover why this exploration is truly a lifelong spiritual practice as we continue to be shaped by our experiences.

This practice of understanding our wholeness and the wholeness of those around us is one which, as Master Xuedou stated, practitioners should not take lightly and only enter into with clear eyes. This work can be difficult, especially at the beginning, but even when we mirror our patients imperfectly, we can still feel the resonance of this type of care. As our practice deepens, this sensitization will increase, allowing for greater validation of the patient's integrity. In this way, spiritual caregivers may help their patients reestablish their identity and internal cohesion, reminding them where they find value in their lives, and returning the agency needed to move toward physical and spiritual healing. How we express our understanding of self and other in relationship each day is our lived response to Master Ma's koan. When truly manifested, there is no chaplain and patient; there is no caregiver and care seeker; there is only Sun Face Buddha, Moon Face Buddha.

I would like to express my appreciation to Sarah M. Peterson for her help in editing this chapter.

16

ICU STAFF ANXIETIES
Originations and Cessations

Acala Xiaoxi Wang

Then Ven. Assaji gave this Dhamma exposition to Sāriputta the Wanderer:
Whatever phenomena arise from cause:
their cause
and their cessation.
Such is the teaching of the Tathagata,
the Great Contemplative.
Then to Sāriputta the wanderer, as he heard this Dhamma exposition,
there arose the dustless, stainless Dhamma eye:
"Whatever is subject to origination is all subject to cessation."

—MAHĀVAGGA 1.23.1–10

"I feel like I'm fighting fires every day." Chaplain Wong leans on a sofa and recalls the words of a chaplain friend who works in a trauma center. How would a chaplain who rushes to fire scenes feel? Will the heat of defilements burst into flames along with the fire of the anxiety of those traumatized families? Tension from a general hospital is indeed not as exhausting as the trauma center. For example, her upcoming 8 p.m. to 8 a.m. night shift at the general hospital usually allows some rest time.

"Ding-ding." The world's never-absent characteristic of impermanence shows through as the text message ringer interrupted Wong's thoughts: "The intensive care unit is experiencing a large increased number of unexpected deaths in recent weeks, and lots of medical staff have become very worried. Please kindly host a fifteen-minute staff support service at the 5 a.m. unit huddle tomorrow morning to help the nurses with transitioning into a new day of work. Appreciated!" The message was sent from a chaplain colleague of that day's day shift staff. It is now approaching the evening. *Suddenly, tomorrow morning,* Wong thinks, *I need to attend to the grieving and anxious medical staff? If I receive other requests to support patients and families during the night, where will I get time to prepare for the morning huddle? After a long night, how can I present a refreshing and full spirit in the morning to bring peace and comfort to the patient care team?*

> There are these three feelings: pleasant feelings, painful feelings, and neither-painful-nor-pleasant feelings. . . . A disciple of the Buddha, mindful, clearly comprehending, with his mind collected, he knows the feelings and their origin, knows whereby they cease, and knows the path that to the ending of feelings lead. And when the end of feelings he has reached, such a monk, his thirsting quenched, attains Nibbāna. —Saṃyutta Nikāya 36.1

The most precious values that a spiritual caregiver can provide to a care receiver are the calm and compassionate presence along with resilience of emotional resonance, so that the care receiver's joy, sorrow, anger, fear, and worry can be expressed unjudged and flow with security. In the process of deep connection with the spiritual caregiver, the care receiver will gradually feel a sense of unconditional self-acceptance and the healing of past trauma. Hence, it is essential to bring a well-balanced mental state from the inside out by the chaplain in a spiritual care service.

> "All conditioned things are impermanent"—when one sees this with wisdom, one turns away from suffering. This is the path to purity.
> Wisdom springs from meditation; without meditation wisdom wanes. Having known these two paths of development and decline, conduct yourself so that wisdom may grow. —Dhammapada 277, 282

After some brief consternation, Wong begins to feel calm. This "fire" does not catch her off guard. From the foundation of daily meditation, a warm current of compassion spontaneously emerged, gently spreading from the bottom of her heart to her entire body, and quickly filled the whole body with an energy of compassion. Wong feels refreshed from the top of her head to the bottom of her feet. To better fulfill tonight's challenge, chaplain Wong gathers herself and sits cross-legged immediately, intending to take advantage of the time left before setting out—she will meditate to further adjust the mind and body to its best state, so as to face the tasks of tonight and the next morning with an energetic, serene, and light spirit. In an emergency situation, the mental preparation of a chaplain is even more important than the planning of service content. For the content, she will primarily rely on her previous accumulation of professional experiences. She hopes and believes that combined with some analysis of the current situation and a calm state of mind, she will be able to adapt to changing conditions around her. The care of the heart is the cornerstone of all wholesome actions as well as the core of people-oriented spiritual care.

> The establishing of mindfulness is to be practiced with the thought, "I'll watch after myself." The establishing of mindfulness is to be practiced with the thought, "I'll watch after others." When watching after yourself, you watch after others. When watching after others, you watch after yourself. And how do you watch after others when watching after yourself? Through cultivating [the practice], through developing it, through pursuing it. This is how you watch after others when watching after yourself. And how do you watch after yourself when watching after others? Through endurance, through harmlessness, through a mind of goodwill, and through empathy. This is how you watch after yourself when watching after others. —Saṃyutta Nikāya 47.19

With a fully renewed sense of faith and energy, Wong comes to the hospital, sits down in front of the computer in the spiritual care office, opens a new document, and begins to create a program for tomorrow's staff support service. Several of the assessments of the situation appear to be particularly critical for a Buddhist chaplain: (1) Given the background of successive deaths of patients, what emotions of the nurses may arise, and what are the corresponding needs? (2) Under the frameworks of chaplaincy theories and Buddhist teachings, what intersection of responses will there be? (3) Considering the natural cycle of emotions, what activities can make the nurses feel seen, empathized, and eventually relieved? (4) The content of interventions must meet the needs of a multifaith or multicultural group and stay within the time limit.

After the assessment outline, the next step is to figure out these questions one by one:

1. Out of responsibility, human nature, and spiritual belief, nurses are likely to experience grief, fear, doubt, anxiety, or depressive moods. These feelings may bring about physical and behavioral changes such as tension, overthinking, loss of motivation, or social isolation. And their corresponding needs could be to relax the body, vent emotions, remember responsibilities, and reconnect with colleagues.

2. The chaplaincy system advocates for the spiritual caregiver to be an empathetic listener and provide a calm presence. By holding space for, witnessing, and normalizing suffering with a care recipient, that person can find something to depend on in the midst of suffering, which in turn develops a broader awareness and understanding of one's individual life. Buddhist texts suggest that people face up to the truth of suffering and its cause through perceiving and contemplating that all worldly phenomena are inconstant, stressful, and not-self. They advocate recognizing, cultivating, and realizing a "right path" that leads to the end of suffering and "right view" is the signpost along the path while concentration and discernment help the vehicle proceed. The intersection of the two is where we must first recognize the existence of the suffering in emotions, and then take a closer assessment of their origination and features. We allow the relief of the body and mind to occur through skillful interventions, so that the spiritual care recipient's ability to discern can be revealed after the grounding of the heart. When this happens, the caretaker's mental state can become more wholesome, and then with a little encouragement, a positive state of mind will be developed toward the responsibilities of the new day.

3. All emotion has a cycle of beginning, developing, transitioning, and ending. Spiritual care must conform to the stages of the emotional cycle to be effective. That is to say, the emotions provoked by the death of patients must first be surfaced, fully validated, and attended to. Activities like making time to honor the deceased, mindfulness exercises for raising self-awareness, or expressing feelings in the group must be performed first. The service can then be supplemented with further

interventions, such as sharing poems or short essays that are directive and inspiring, and finally encouraging self-care or team activities with interpersonal connection at the end.

4. Due to the limited time of this service, and the estimated large number of participants, after difficult consideration, a session where nurses take turns speaking and exchanging feelings was dropped, even though generally speaking, such sessions are very beneficial to calm the mood and generate a collective sense of belonging. In contrast, this particular service event focuses on letting feelings touch base with the realities of life by listening to a piece of prose. Through this, nurses will extend their perspective from the single event of the death of a patient to looking at the entire life process and meaning throughout the past and present. The goals are (a) to achieve acceptance and normalization of the occurrence of deaths by broadening the horizon, (b) finding a balance between controllable and uncontrollable in the process of imagining the universality and limitations of the roles played by themselves and their patients in their long history, (c) establishing faith and confidence in matters within their competence, and (4) starting care for their patients and colleagues again with a renewed sense of vitality in their work.

And how is right view the forerunner? In one of right view, right resolve comes into being. In one of right resolve, right speech comes into being. In one of right speech, right action. . . . In one of right action, right livelihood. . . . In one of right livelihood, right effort. . . . In one of right effort, right mindfulness. . . . In one of right mindfulness, right concentration. . . . In one of right concentration, right knowledge. . . . In one of right knowledge, right release comes into being. —Majjhima Nikāya 117

Wong cannot help smiling as she looks through the service plan in front of her: despite containing a meditation-inspired method for soothing the mind and body, a reflection prose written on the basis of a Buddhist discourse, and an interactive activity designed to bless nursing colleagues with the concept of loving-kindness as the core, none of them goes against the basic principle by which an interfaith spiritual caregiver should always abide: to be respectful and inclusive of all beliefs. Every participant can see themselves from this service program regardless of which belief system they identify with or what insight they have into life. Although it may still be far from perfect, it is a solid plan that Wong is able to come up with under time constraints. The composition is timely, factual, and situational. During the process of creating this service program, Wong received two urgent requests to depart for the ward, and it is past three in the morning by the time she finishes writing the program. Fortunately, the meditation practice prior to this shift energized her. Now Wong only feels compassion in her heart without any sense of exhaustion. She feels that with just a short break, she will be able to head to the intensive care unit before 5 a.m. for the huddle.

> For one whose awareness-release through good will is cultivated, developed, pursued, handed the reins and taken as a basis, given a grounding, steadied, consolidated, and well-undertaken, eleven benefits can be expected. Which eleven?
>
> One sleeps easily, wakes easily, dreams no evil dreams. One is dear to human beings, dear to nonhuman beings. The devas protect one. Neither fire, poison, nor weapons can touch one. One's mind gains concentration quickly. One's complexion is bright. One dies unconfused and—if penetrating no higher—is headed for the Brahma worlds. —Aṅguttara Nikāya 11.16

4:45 a.m. Wong tidies up her clothes, clips on the badge, puts on the mask and safety goggles, takes her work phone and the staff support program sheet, and sets off for the intensive care unit. The corridor of the hospital is very quiet in the morning. Only a few medical staff are walking under the fluorescent ceiling light along the way, and soon Wong arrives at the destination. Following the double door and walking straight in, passing several closed office doors on both sides, turning left after approaching the large brass characters of "Intensive Care Unit" on the cream-colored wall, in less than ten steps Wong sees the nurse station where the huddle will be held. The nurse station is in the center of the unit, mainly constructed by a circle of desks and chairs that enables a broad field of vision over the ward. There are some medical staff sitting and standing beside the monitors on the desk inside the station. Among them is a woman arranging patient care plans for two other nurses with the definite tone of someone in charge. She is in a flannel jacket with the hospital logo, appearing easygoing yet authoritative. As soon as her conversation is over, Wong steps forward to greet her, introduce herself, and explain the reason for the visit. This woman is indeed the charge nurse. She warmly welcomes Wong and confirms the arrangement of the staff support service.

Within only a few minutes, the nurse station is surrounded by layers of medical staff. About forty people attend the huddle. The charge nurse and Wong are in the center of the crowd. At 5 a.m. sharp, seeing the confirmation from the charge nurse, Wong introduces herself and conveys her concern for everyone in a gentle and firm tone, and then the service formally begins. First, Wong invites everyone to participate in a minute of silence, to acknowledge the grief and honor the deceased, and to pay respect to each other's hard work to provide the best care possible for the patients. Nurses who are chatting in low voices quiet down, everyone stands silently with their eyes closed and their heads down, the atmosphere in the unit becomes noticeably solemn. When the minute is up, Wong asks everyone to open their eyes, soften their sights, gently embrace their own bodies with two arms, and listen to this guidance, which she strives to speak in a soothing tone:

> Hugging myself, I allow my heart to feel
> the grief, sorrow, fear, and heaviness.
> Hugging myself, I allow my body to feel
> the warmth, security, comfort, and relief.
> Hugging myself, I allow my mind to feel
> centered, calm, easeful, and compassionate.

Wong then pauses in silence for a moment, watching everyone immersed in their respective emotions, then begins using a slow rhythm to read the prose she prepared earlier, guiding the nurses to reflect upon the truths of life:

> The circle of life and death started 3.5 billion years ago when our Earth had her first tiny living being. Without pause since then is this miracle of birth, living, illness, and death. Time after time. On every corner of this planet, throughout the river of history till tomorrow, living and dying are happening. When life is brief, fragile, and uncertain, what gives it meaning? What sustains me and what do I live for? Maybe because my parents wanted to express their love for me; maybe because I wanted to love my loved ones; maybe because I have passion for experiencing an adventurous journey; maybe because I wish to care for the sick and their families; or maybe because I have a vocation to serve a higher power or achieve an actualization. So do

my patients. They experienced a purpose. They made a legacy. Every person's
will or soul is a thread of energy that can never be increased or destroyed.
When one finishes one's task on Earth, one's existence transforms and reap-
pears somewhere else, in our memory, in nature, for some beliefs, in another
womb, in heaven. But I know, today, I am here. Still, a patient may die, just
like an ancestor died a hundred years ago. I let go of what is not in my control
and say my farewell. A survivor may grieve; I say my comforting words and
gently lend my hands. I will do what I can. I will take care of myself and wish
that everyone around me be healthy and happy.

After reading the whole prose, Wong senses that the nurses' moods grew signifi-
cantly calmer, and she knows it is time to rebuild the team spirit. Wong reminds
the nurses that one of the best ways to cope with uneasiness and loneliness is to
generously spread goodwill to those around them. Everyone is invited to pair
up, look into each other's eyes with a genuine smile, and take turns to say a few
words of gratitude or blessing. For example, one can say: "Thank you for the
care you give, the healing you provide, and the work you do. I wish you a safe,
smooth, and joyful day." When the nurses hear this instruction, they all glance
at their colleagues with a shy look. Indeed, in the midst of our busy schedule, do
we often neglect to express our care and appreciation for those who are standing beside us in our lives? Although the staff appears to be a little uncertain at
first, the hesitation is soon overwhelmed by a sudden wave of laughter with each
other. Everyone is moved by the person beside them and sharing sincere wishes
that only those who are in the same situation can understand. The staff support service concludes on time with a warm and pleasant atmosphere. Affected
by the uplifting emotions of each nurse and the heartfelt connections among
them, Wong feels others' trust and can go to the cafeteria for breakfast with
peace of mind.

> These four are to be known as friends who are loyal: One who is helpful is to
> be known as a friend who is loyal. One who is pleased and pained together
> with you is to be known as a friend who is loyal. One who points out your
> benefit is to be known as a friend who is loyal. One who is empathetic is to be
> known as a friend who is loyal. —Dīgha Nikāya 31

*The story for this chapter is adapted from personal experiences as a chaplain in
an ICU.*

17

BUDDHAS IN THE MEDICAL INTENSIVE CARE UNIT

Reflecting a Workspace in the Mandala

Stephanie Barnes (Repa Nyima Ozer)

"Room three just died; you can start there." My first instruction, on my first day, as a chaplain in training. It was delivered from a charge nurse, in a monotone voice, as she remained glued to her computer screen in the busy emergency room of a small upstate New York hospital. I told the nurse, "OK," and headed for the staff locker room to hang up my coat. After I placed it on a hook, a string of obscenities exited my mouth in a whisper as I strived to reach for breath, prayer, for the Buddhas, bodhisattvas, gods, angels, *dakas, dakinis;* whoever might be listening.

Twenty-three years prior, I brought my two-year-old son to this same emergency room in the middle of the night. I had stood next to his hospital gurney as an emergency room physician told me that he did not think my son would make it. The emotion of that moment washed over me as I gathered myself to attend to the situation in room three. Thankfully, my son survived, but that memory turned up the intensity of the emergency room. Thinking of that night—along with moving toward a room with a dead body, and probably a distraught family—felt overwhelming. My Dharma training felt both present *and* distant, but I managed to connect to my breath, put my head up and shoulders down, and then I drew back the curtain. My childhood conditioning trained me to look confident despite enormous internal fear. At this moment, it provided ground on which to stand. I don't remember the prayer I offered with the family of the deceased, but I remember being present, making eye contact, and listening to their pain to the best of my ability. When I left the hospital that day, I knew I would need to find a way to stabilize my mind, my breath, my body. Because I am a Vajrayāna Buddhist practitioner and an artist, visualization provided the stability I needed. At my next shift, when I arrived at the hospital steps, I paused and mentally removed my shoes, made three bows, offered an aspiration prayer, and entered the building the way I would a shrine or zendo. Treating the hospital as sacred space was just what I needed, reminding me to bring everything I encounter onto the path.

Several years later, as a chaplain resident in a Level 1 trauma center and teaching hospital, I was asked to choose which block of units I wanted to cover during my residency. My supervisor had organized sections of the hospital into blocks. Each one included five to seven units of the trauma center. My Dharma teacher is the head of chaplaincy for the City of New York's Department of Corrections, so I was inspired to choose the block with the locked prison unit. That block also included infectious diseases, the neurological ICU, the hospitalist unit, and the medical intensive care unit (MICU). I had very little sense of what the units would entail, outside of the prison unit. I was excited, scared, and so focused on getting the prison unit that I did not think to inquire further about what the MICU actually was. I was to learn pretty fast: over the next nine months, I would attend an average of four to six deaths per day, most of them in the MICU.

As my residency unfolded, I became aware of the sensations in my body when I was paged to the MICU. My pulse became rapid, my breath shallow, my mind and thoughts more accelerated. This was not surprising: I was facing terminal extubations, deaths, drug overdoses, alcohol poisoning, families in crisis, violent eruptions between family members, people at odds with each other and within themselves while confronting decisions to remove life support or to continue extraordinary measures. Chaplains find themselves in the middle of it all, holding space as a nonanxious presence, witnessing, reflecting, steadying the air.

To calm my own physical reactions, one of the first things I tried was standing like a superhero in the elevators on my way to calls: face to the sky, hands on hips, feet planted apart in defiance of any arising fear. This exercise provided a strange and silly kind of confidence until I noticed the security cameras in the corners of the elevators. The idea of anyone reviewing the camera footage and coming upon the chaplain impersonating Wonder Woman in the elevator brought much needed laughter to my fellow chaplaincy residents.

One practice I did develop as the calls for me to respond to the MICU increased was reciting mantra as I moved through the hospital corridors, allowing my mind to rest, my body to relax, and my breath to steady.

I came to understand that the medical team on the unit must also be holding enormous tension in their bodies. I had learned in my first smaller hospital that staff appreciated and valued the guided meditation I introduced. I adapted this practice for the MICU to help doctors and nurses gain confidence and skill in using their breath to remain grounded and supported, no matter what was unfolding. Quite naturally, staff in intensive care units often feel unable or unwilling to leave their post to attend meditation or prayer groups. I began to sit one-on-one or in small clusters to help the medical team connect to their breath while in the trauma and chaos of the moment. Over time, staff reported that just seeing this chaplain enter the MICU gave them peace and reminded them to turn to their breath without much thought. The impromptu daily meditation sessions became a staple in the MICU and have become an important part of my Buddhist ministry.

In Vajrayāna Buddhism, the "Diamond Vehicle" or "Thunderbolt Vehicle," one uses tantric practice to enact Buddhist ideals—transmuting ordinary perception into sacred outlook as one wishes enlightenment for the benefit of all sentient beings. Transforming the mind undergirds all Buddhist practice, and I value the fact that chaplaincy takes that experience *off* the cushion and into action. As the weeks went by, I began to view the MICU as sacred space and all its inhabitants as Buddhas. I saw the similarity between the physical layout of an intensive care unit and a Buddhist mandala. Both are squares with four gates containing a circle with a center point or palace; a mandala's purpose is to transform the mind and bring healing. So too an ICU, with its nurses station at its center, surrounded by rows of rooms on four sides like protective barriers, entrances from its corners, oriented to the four quarters of the world, all surrounded by outlying charnel grounds. The formation naturally lends itself to the circular motion of *kora,* or circumambulation, on foot or in the mind through visualization, while summoning the qualities of the deity associated with the mandala. While the staff was not Buddhist themselves, my own engagement with the space as mandala provided me stability, peace, and centeredness. This in turn provided support and stability to staff, patients, and their loved ones in this highly charged environment, and the concept could be used on any hospital unit where I ministered.

In my last weeks with the MICU staff, a nurse told me how much she had appreciated what I brought to the team, noting how at first, the meditation had felt foreign and strange in these circumstances, but that it had become an incredibly valued and intrinsic part of their day.

As I prepared to say good-bye to the doctors and nurses of the MICU, I designed and made a large *tankha* to hang on the wall in the MICU staff room. The tankha depicted a mandala, honoring the dedicated work of the MICU team. Outside a large ring of red cloth, depicting fire, each of the five Buddha families were represented by their colors: blue for Akshobhya, representing patience; yellow for Ratnasambhava, equanimity; red for Amitābha, compassion; green for Amogasiddha, joy; and white for Vairocana, wisdom. The four corners were red, blue, green, and yellow. The center was a large white pocket in which I put small ribbons in red, blue, green, yellow, and white with safety pins. Staff were encouraged to help themselves to a ribbon to pin on their lapel. Next to the tankha was a key listing the virtue associated with each color. I encouraged staff to pick a ribbon and pin it to their lapel each day, keeping the virtue in mind.

When I entered the MICU the day after hanging the tankha, staff members proudly displayed the ribbon they had chosen and shouted out for me to see their lapels, many telling me of the feeling of confidence it gave them. I smiled and my heart beamed as I silently continued the mantra of the deity I had chosen for this mandala. I should mention here that traditionally, each of the poisons would also be noted along with the virtues (white: ignorance, blue: aggression, yellow: pride, red: passion or grasping, green: jealously). However, I intentionally chose to omit the poisons from the key of colors. In my experience, nurses and doctors working in this kind of intense atmosphere are extremely hard on themselves and benefit from the offer to focus on what they did well.

Since leaving that residency, I have worked in a prison and home hospice. As of 2020, I am an EMS chaplain and hospital chaplain in a trauma center in northern New Mexico on a COVID unit, aspiring to bring it all to the path.

The mandala, and all of its transformative wisdom qualities, is a useful object both in physical form and in visualization—vast, available, and limitless as space itself. Impromptu meditation is often the only form of meditation possible in hospital settings, and my own visualization during a shift has remained a mainstay and helped me to continue to be of service during unprecedented times.

18

EXPERIMENTS IN MINDFULNESS

A Collaborative Health-Care Staff Support Program

Shushin R. A. Peterson

I was serving as a hospital chaplain resident when COVID-19 arrived in force in March 2020. As public health restrictions went into effect, all but essential staff were sent to work from home, and our hospital entered a time of anxiety and uncertainty. Chaplains are considered essential workers and so we continued to arrive and serve our now isolated inpatient community. As increasing signs of compassion fatigue and other forms of emotional distress appeared, a dedicated care team was established to implement resiliency programs to aid our staff in an ongoing pandemic environment. One of the programs this team created was called the Stress-Management Mindfulness Series, spearheaded by our health system's psychologists.

The Stress-Management Mindfulness Series

As a Buddhist chaplain within the Sōtō Zen tradition, I was invited to participate in leading the series, and I was the only self-identified Buddhist on the team. Mindfulness is featured heavily in many psychological modalities, and its use as a secular tool for grounding and stress relief has become fairly cemented within Western clinical care. The Stress-Management Mindfulness Series offered daily ten- to fifteen-minute call-in sessions where team members would rotate in leading participants through various mindfulness exercises. To decrease distractions, there was no interaction among participants, nor were webcams used for our online participants. Contact information for questions or concerns was provided via email, and the series ran daily for about six months.

Overall, reception of the program was very positive. Participants expressed appreciation for a dedicated moment of self-care each day during a period of increased stress as well as reporting feelings of increased social connection during a period of physical isolation. We gathered a small core of participants who called in daily within a larger fluctuating audience, including participants from other hospitals within our health-care system. Due to the positive feedback the program received, hospital leadership decided to retain the Mindfulness Series as a permanent resiliency program and transform it into a yearly training framework for social work and psychology interns.

Given my own experience with mindfulness in a religious rather than secular setting, I was excited to see this level of enthusiasm for mindfulness within our hospital. I also encountered several noteworthy differences in the presentation of mindfulness. I will use the terms *Buddhist* and *secular* to discuss the differences in practice and orientation that I observed throughout the series, though many of the specific exercises used by both Buddhists and secular clinicians are similar, and not all Buddhist traditions utilize mindfulness as a spiritual practice. *Secular* will refer to the practices and underlying assumptions about the mind in Western psychological and social-work disciplines. Our series was designed for those with little exposure to meditative practice, and with only ten- to fifteen-minute sessions, the deeper subtleties and diversity of Buddhist practices were not fully explored. Within these limitations, I refer to the nonsecular practices in the series as "Buddhist" for the purpose of this discussion, even though this term is an overgeneralization for a discussion taking place solely within my tradition. The following comments are based on my own direct experiences and engagement with my colleagues during the series. Mental health disciplines may have other modalities that address the Buddhist themes I discuss, and if so, I hope the following comments can be used for further interdisciplinary collaboration between Buddhist religious practitioners and mental health professionals.

As the series progressed, I discovered that the differences between Buddhist and secular practices stemmed from both within the mindfulness exercises themselves and from our underlying orientations toward mindfulness in general. The following discussion of these differences will broaden into a further exploration of the orientations behind Buddhist and secular assumptions of the mind and reality. I will then conclude with how these differences may facilitate future opportunities for collaboration in similar projects. Through such collaboration, some of the original flavor and orientation of Buddhist practices that have been secularized may be regained and further utilized in offering care to those we serve both in times of crisis and in overall support of our community's well-being.

Differences in Buddhist and Secular Practice

The largest difference between Buddhist and secular mindfulness practice to emerge from our series centered on the role of this-moment awareness of the body. Many of the secular practices focused almost exclusively on physical awareness through body scans. For instance, session leaders would instruct participants to "Focus on your feet and the sensation of them resting on the floor." These practices occasionally expanded into relaxation where points of pain or tension were intentionally released. There are Buddhist techniques that focus on pure physicality within the concentration family of meditation practice, but when these were presented from the Buddhist perspective during the series, they held underlying encouragement to explore the foundational doctrine of emptiness. This encouragement was sometimes through direct instruction to watch bodily sensations rise and fall with the understanding that those sensations are not part of a concrete self. This utilized the techniques taught in body-based Satipatthana (scriptural mindfulness practices), while other explorations of emptiness came through more subtly, such as simple vocabulary shifts from "observe your feet" to simply "observe the feet."

Buddhist practices also extended beyond the physical during the series, exploring deeper Buddhist doctrines and values. These practices included exploring the four *brahmavihārās* of kindness, compassion, joy, and equanimity, and the interconnection and mutual support between each of these four practices. Kindness and compassion practices included focused *mettā* and Tonglen practice. Mettā practices focused on offering goodwill to both oneself and others. The more active compassion practice of Tonglen involved a visualized intake of suffering while responding with specific offerings of care for that suffering. Instruction on supporting the interplay between the brahmavihārās was also explored, such as balancing compassion and compassion fatigue with equanimity, and the optimism of joy was embodied through offerings of kindness.

Different flavors of traditional teaching methods within Buddhism were presented, such as "holding a question," often used as an introduction to koan practice in Chan (Zen) traditions. In this practice, a question is asked, such as "Who am I?" and all conceptual responses to that question are intentionally deconstructed. Minor techniques for addressing hindrances were also presented. One technique involved noting points of physical or emotional discomfort. Rather than shifting position or stopping one's practice, the unpleasant sensations became an intentional offering with internalized phrases such as "May this pain be the pain of all sentient beings, so they need not suffer it." Other minor techniques included Master Zhiyi's sound syllables for calming the heart, where a single sound is uttered for the entirety of one's exhalation while simultaneously massaging the chest.

The next major difference between secular and Buddhist styles focused on the role of inherent or universal morality. Before this difference is addressed directly, a few comments should be made about the underlying orientations of Buddhist and Western psychology. The foundations of this difference lie in *who* is making these moral decisions. Assuming an underlying self or ego for much of Western psychological history, secular practices in the series tended to focus on how this self relates with itself and other factors in the environment, most notably the body. The Buddhist doctrines of emptiness and no-self, on the other hand, present the self as a continual flux of mutually dependent parts without an ultimate substance. Harvey Aronson, author of *Buddhist Practice on Western Ground,* outlines these two psychological orientations with far more detail and precision than is possible here, and is highly recommended for those interested in this topic. Aronson concludes that this divergence results in a difference of emphasis between *process* and *content* when examining the mind. Western psychology focuses on content, or how the ego defines its inherent autonomy and relates and adapts to its surroundings and other inherent actors. Buddhist teachings focus on process, examining how the interactions studied by Western psychology rise and fall, appear and disappear, and, through deeper spiritual practice, hopefully lead to a spiritual awakening.

This underlying divergence was not explored during the series, but it was clearly present in the language used during the exercises. A common secular practice upheld the self as an inherent actor through visualizing a stream, with the instructions that "*you* place *your* thoughts on leaves and watch them float away, leaving *you* free from distraction." Buddhist practices, as discussed above, emphasized a greater orientation toward the rise and fall of bodily and mental fabrications, cultivation of values, and questions about our own self-nature, holding the implicit assumption of emptiness, or mutual interconnection, as the underlying nature of reality.

After noting these differences in Buddhist and Western assumptions about the true nature of the self, we can return to the different assumptions about morality found in the series. If there is an inherent nature to reality, then there are inherent methods that help or hinder our realization of these truths, and these methods can be framed as moral practice. A basic secular assumption within the series, however, was that each individual is the source of their own value structure, something that many chaplains would agree with. For example, some patients might uphold relationships more than institutions, or intellectual knowledge more than emotional understanding. During the occasional non-bodily-based secular practice, a person's own value system was often blurred to operate as an objective moral system, such as when a religious devotee presents deepening faith as objective knowledge. Buddhist tradition, however, upholds an inherent moral system removed from personal preference.

While moral systems in Buddhism are more nuanced than this statement implies, all traditions present versions of the same precepts, founded in the same basic values of caring for life, compassion for others, and guarding one's behavior to prevent physical, emotional, or spiritual harm to oneself or others. Even the relativism implied by *upāya* or "skillful means" in Mahāyāna Buddhism requires a deeper objective moral orientation of how our actions ultimately impact suffering. With roots in the Noble Eightfold Path, there are objective moral understandings within Buddhism that may be at odds with an individual's internal values. While both secular and Buddhist approaches attempt to work with an individual's already established value system, secular exercises during the series tended to stop at awareness and did not question the validity of the practitioners' assumptions about value or meaning in their lives. There was some discussion by members of the leadership team that what a general audience might consider "good" or "bad" would naturally reveal itself through only engaging in secular awareness; however there was no active challenge to any preconceived values in the series.

Outside the series, morality is a foundation of Buddhist mindfulness through both concentration and wisdom practices, as they attempt to guide us along varying routes of personal reflection about our actions and their consequences in order to show us the roots of our suffering. Concentration practices, which were mostly what the series focused on, teach practitioners the ability to hold a single point in focus without distraction. Concentration upholds wisdom practices, especially when focusing on distressing topics, such as our imminent mortality or examining how our actions have caused harm in the past. To face these aspects of our existence requires that we are neither piling on new suffering from unethical actions or being lured by sensual pleasures and other distractions to avoid the reality of our situation. This type of journey requires a backing of objective morality much like a tomato cage supports the vine as it grows upward. As practice continues, realization of the relief of coming to terms with past actions and the liberation of not creating new scenarios of suffering emerges. In this way, Buddhist wisdom practices demonstrate the objective validity of values such as generosity and gratitude or the dangers of hatred and delusion.

A natural extension of this difference of moral viewpoint, implied but not explicit during our series, is the role of orienting our entire life toward specific values. In most secular practices, very few fundamental changes in our life need to be enacted. If a person values wealth, sensual pleasure, or power, then secular mindfulness practices allow them to orient more fully toward these values as they develop the ability to put down distraction and create space to act, rather than react. In terms of how Buddhism understands suffering and the cessation of suffering, validating personal values like those listed above would create great difficulties in leading someone to peace, let alone spiritual awakening.

Buddhist practices operate from the assumption that mindfulness is performed within the framework of a life guided by the objective values of the Noble Eightfold Path. Regardless of how aware we are, if we carry a wrong view, engage in wrong effort toward unwholesome goals, or perform wrong actions when off the cushion, no amount of mindfulness will alleviate our ultimate distress. Mindfulness unhinged from this moral backing has been used at certain points in Buddhist history, most notably within my own tradition during World War II in the support of military aggression, creating a legacy of suffering that we are still addressing today. On a smaller scale, without a moral backing, mindfulness would help blanket feelings of guilt when cutting corners at work, or uphold disinterest or detachment when implementing policies that directly harm the well-being of others, such as reducing salaries, sick leave, or other benefits. In these situations, mindfulness will help individuals soothe internal resistance to such actions in the moment, but it will not erase the harm that might come about from such actions or help remove the deeper attachments that prompted such actions in the first place. Mirroring the Buddhist doctrine of emptiness, any effective mindfulness practice can only exist within an interconnected relationship of mutual support with all aspects of the Noble Eightfold Path.

This distinction between practice and daily life also highlights another core pan-Buddhist teaching that neither the Buddhist nor secular practices in the series were able to fully implement. Mindfulness as a spiritual practice is one that must extend beyond a specific exercise. When beginning a spiritual mindfulness practice, it is difficult to have awareness of the body, let alone an awareness of how the mind is engaging with internal and external stimuli in the present moment. There are too many distractions vying for our attention. Practice therefore starts in a quiet room for a limited time, not because this is the whole of practice, but because this is the limit of concentration for many beginners. As practice deepens, we learn to hold our mindfulness even with increased activity and distraction.

One area that helps bridge mindfulness meditation and the activities of daily life is ritual. Ritual provides a clear structure to evaluate one's own actions since ritual actions are performed the same way each time. This allows participants a clearer understanding of when their minds are distracted or hooked by other concerns that are identified by variations within one's ritual performance. For example, if there is no standard for brushing one's teeth, it becomes more difficult to understand if the hurried or relaxed way that it might manifest on any given day is the result of inattention, preoccupation, or intentional focus. Leading a ritualized life both within religious communities and at home creates guideposts. These allow practitioners to expand mindfulness practice farther into daily life and help more clearly identify challenges that may arise when proactively exploring and engaging the mind and its processes.

This expansion of mindful action into all aspects of daily life was not possible within the confines of the series for either secular or Buddhist practices. Secular practices were presented as definitive in terms of content and time, while Buddhist practices could do no more than offer encouragement to extend one's period of mindful intention and attention forward throughout the day. Without the gradual extension of mindfulness to all actions throughout the day, any mindfulness practice falls into the same dangers outlined above regarding the eroding impact of unwholesome action on one's practice.

A final area of difference between secular and Buddhist mindfulness resides in the limited potential of simple awareness. Secular practices presented this-moment awareness as the end goal of mindfulness. Buddhist practices in the series always ended with an injunction to use any developed calmness or clarity to make proactive choices in the future. Awareness is only the gateway to deeper understanding. Awareness can only be useful if it eventually operates in conjunction with both past memory and future intention. Substantial present-moment awareness may be needed to know what our current situation actually is, or to understand how our past choices brought us here, but this clarity is not the final goal. After we clearly see where we are now, both mentally and physically, the next step of future intention can be applied. How do we wish to respond to similar situations in the future?

When all three parts of mindfulness work together—clarity of memory, present-moment awareness, and future intention—we finally arrive at the freedom to respond in either similar or different ways to the situations we encounter. Depending on one's Buddhist tradition, this process may be similar to that outlined above, or have a greater emphasis on spontaneous realization gained through engaging these questions in nonconceptual practice. Many secular practices in the series acknowledged the space between stimuli, action, and reaction, which awareness helps us find, but how we direct our intention once this space is discovered was not addressed and left entirely to each participant's relative perspective. Buddhist practices, in contrast, would not leave such choices to personal discretion; they have very clear guidance on which responses should be cultivated.

Opportunities for Future Collaboration

The differences outlined between secular and Buddhist orientations toward mindfulness present opportunities for collaboration between Buddhist religious professionals and those from other disciplines. Using a similar secular mindfulness series as a framework, there are several areas in which a Buddhist understanding of mindfulness could support resiliency among an organization's staff or patient population.

My experience with the series indicated that mindfulness presented from a secular viewpoint was fully proficient in teaching and upholding the Buddhist skills of present-moment awareness, understanding of the mind-body relationship, and assisting in relaxation or stress reduction. All of these are introductory skills that many Buddhists cultivate within their own practice. Through collaboration, these introductory practices, presented in a secular format, can guide a wider audience, and as proficiency develops, there is an opportunity to transition into more overt spiritual practices, extending the spiritual, emotional, and mental cultivation that has already begun.

The first area that might be informed by Buddhist practices is in the realm of objective values. Without making overt truth claims during a series, Buddhist practices could orient toward assumptions of the objective value in generosity, gratitude, or the relief that comes when operating without an emphasis on self. Buddhist practices could also be used to explore a more fundamental understanding of cause and effect, as well as attachment as a source of suffering. These ideas could be introduced simply as concluding remarks at the end of a ten-minute session, encouraging attendees to remain aware and intentional in their actions toward specific values, such as the brahmavihārās (lovingkindness, compassion, joy, and equanimity). Values could also be addressed broadly, by creating thematic phases within a long-term program that devotes one or two weeks of daily practice to a specific value, such as compassion. Another option would be the intentional cultivation of the desire to practice, such as those outlined in the scripture Encouragement to Giving Rise to the Bodhi Mind. With these basic values-based assumptions, Buddhist practices can encourage the exploration of areas of life outside of mindfulness sessions and assist in developing an understanding of how our daily choices impact our experience of stress and well-being.

Buddhist responses to this full-life orientation are reflected in the importance of the Sangha, a community of both support and fellow practitioners. The series offered a reflection of this community as we joined together each day. However, it was not cohesive in terms of orientation, purpose, and understanding of practice, nor was it in person. Creating more explicit support groups geared directly toward mindfulness practices through either secular or explicitly Buddhist frameworks may be another area of collaboration. Focused on mindfulness, such groups would have the potential to expand into the realm of social support and fellowship. Although it would not be able to replace the deeper bond and roles of the Sangha, such a group would allow the encouragement and security offered by the Sangha to be more manifest in the lives of series members. These deeper interactions with the group would also allow opportunities to explore ways in which ritual or mindful action could be extended into other activities of daily life, such as mindfulness exercises focused on eating or drinking, melding with values work focused on gratitude or appreciation.

Religious professionals should be aware that some secular clinicians may identify as Buddhists themselves. In these situations, Buddhist clinicians often have a better understanding and appreciation of Buddhist religious professionals. The role of professional ethics places limits on how manifest one's personal beliefs can be when operating as a health-care professional in a mental-health or social-work role. The role of chaplaincy, however, allows Buddhist religious professionals to fully bring their tradition with them when presenting mindfulness techniques. Ordained Buddhist chaplains also bring a deeper understanding of how all aspects of Buddhist practice inform and uphold each other, as well as an understanding of the limits of individual practices when they are stripped from the supportive framework of their parent tradition. When Buddhists are able to collaborate with other health-care and mental health professionals in this way, it provides the opportunity for all present to experience some of the flavor and nuance that has been lost as mindfulness transitioned into a secular practice.

This holistic life application points to a last, deeper theme that influences both secular and Buddhist forms of mindfulness practice. Most health-care professionals who use mindfulness tend to focus on individual issues, disorders, or traumas. Overarching themes within one's life are usually not addressed, except insofar as they impact a specific event or diagnosis. As discussed above, the interconnection of our existence and the mutuality present in the different aspects of full Buddhist practice all focus on the integration of this practice with all other aspects of our life. Such total integrative work is not available through many secular approaches to mindfulness. The series itself was presented as a response to a supposedly specific and isolated event, the COVID-19 pandemic, instead of as a program to support our staff's overall orientation toward their lives. However, as the hospital staff received our offering, there was subtle acknowledgment of the interconnection between the mindfulness practices and the lives of the participants, extending beyond the pandemic as a specific point of crisis. This acknowledgment came in the form of establishing the series as a permanent program that can uphold and improve many people's well-being, regardless of circumstance.

To see mindfulness practices taking on a greater role and acceptance within formalized health-care settings is greatly encouraging. I was impressed by my own hospital's willingness to offer such a program to our staff, and the experience has been greatly rewarding. As we develop future mindfulness programming, opportunities for collaboration and deeper integration of Buddhist tradition more explicitly as Buddhist tradition will appear as well. Through mutual support and professional respect, Buddhists have ever-widening opportunities to work with other clinicians toward the holistic mental and spiritual health of our community.

I would like to express my appreciation to Sarah M. Peterson for her help in editing this chapter.

19

CHAPLAINS NEED CHAPLAINS TOO

Chenxing Han

❖

Three-quarters of the way into my yearlong residency in hospital chaplaincy, I figure I've finally gotten a handle on spiritual care. I've had a twenty-four-hour on-call shift every week for the past nine months. I'm confident I can handle anything the unpredictable nights have to offer.

And then comes the call that blasts my confidence asunder.

❖

I am paged by a nurse to come and support "a few distraught family members" for "a patient who is expiring." Upon arriving at the ICU, I realize that "a few" means about fifteen (how did they all fit into this tiny room?), "distraught" is code for complete pandemonium, and "expiring" can now be rendered in the past tense. It is like walking onto a stage where the apogees of a dozen gut-wrenching plays are happening simultaneously.

My first instinct is to flee. Two men stand dazed outside the door.

The nurse sees me and gasps with relief, "Oh, good, you're the chaplain."

I may have muttered, "Oh, shit," under my breath at this point.

Inside the cramped room, men and women are crying, beating their bodies, stomping, howling. They are shouting in a language I will later learn is Tigre, one of the nine national languages of Eritrea. Someone is thrashing around on the floor.

On the bed, a thin woman with braided hair is dead. Her neck is bent to the left. A thin line of blood trails from her mouth to the pillow. She looks younger than the age listed in her medical chart, so much so that I mistake one of her daughters for a sister. This daughter is screaming in rage, kicking the floor, being restrained by two family members. Another young woman leans against a dripping faucet, cradling her head, still as a statue. A third woman is pounding her chest and legs in a trance, chanting, "oo-wee, oo-wee, oo-wee"— or is it, "oh, why, oh, why, oh, why?"

More family come. Fresh wails erupt. All around me people are moving and people are collapsing, people are hyperventilating, and people are retching. The noise level is deafening.

Even the seasoned ICU nurses are panicked, tears pricking their eyes as they ask, "What should we do?" They beg me to calm everyone down. I am feeling inadequate, inadequate, inadequate.

In a room of chaos, one calm person makes a difference.

In a room of chaos, one calm person might not stay calm for long.

This might have been a good time to call in reinforcements.

One of the daughters gestures to me and then points at her mother's body. "Do you see her? She was the *best mother* in the *world. Why did she have to die? Why?!*"

"What are your favorite memories of her?" As soon as the words escape my mouth, I silently rebuke myself. This is a later question, not a now question. It's too soon. Later there will be time for remembrance. Now she is gripped in holy war with her mother's gone-ness.

"There are no words for my mother. No words!" she shrieks.

There is no fairy dust I can sprinkle on this situation to get everyone to magically settle down. Our imperfect tools—word, song, chant, ablution, prayer beads, smudge of soot, dab of oil—we use them all, but even the most resourceful chaplain cannot escape the moment when everything in her toolbox fails.

A thin young woman—nose piercing, sweatpants, I have to reduce the cast to the barest of identifying details to keep track—stumbles as if drunk, drapes herself over the body on the bed. An older man tries to remove her.

"No! Let me go! Don't!"

"Don't act like this. I am going to take you home."

"No!"

"It won't be finished in a day."

The daughter who is kicking the floor points an accusatory finger at the ceiling.

"I was the *strong* one when she was alive," she shouts. "I *fought* for her; I was *strong* for her. *She gave up on me.* How could she?!"

This storm will not be stifled. I act on adrenaline, hew to simplicity. Make sure no one gets hurt. Coax saltines and juice boxes into the mouths of those who are close to fainting. Gather everyone for a brief attempt at prayer. Watch the scene fragment back into chaos. Bow to the magnitude and endurance of a maelstrom that shows no sign of abating.

•

My introduction to Buddhist chaplaincy came six years prior to this maelstrom. That summer, I witness the skillful compassion of the staff members of Brahmavihara, an NGO founded in Phnom Penh, Cambodia, by Reverend Beth Kanji Goldring to offer spiritual care for the gravely ill and dying. Knowing barely a word of Cambodian, confronted with more sickness and death in those couple of months than in the span of my twenty-two years up to that point, I learn the inadequacy of my newly minted undergraduate degree.

That summer, on a trip to the Phnom Penh countryside, I meet Koet Ran, a beloved Cambodian Dharma song *(smot)* master who teaches the intricate melodies and multilayered narratives that make smot such a haunting and powerful form of music. She greets me as she does each of her grandchildren: with a grin so wide her blind eyes crease shut, with warm palms that cradle every contour of my smiling face. Koet Ran has over thirty grandchildren, and she can distinguish every one with a loving caress of the cheek as surely as she can sing scores of Dharma songs from memory.

It can take hours to perform just one of these sacred songs. A single line can take three minutes. Koet Ran teaches me the opening of "Orphan's Lament."[1] I run out of air before reaching the second word.

It's the song I wish I could have sung to the Eritrean family.

Woe, woe! I'm now an orphan
I'm broken without Mother
All alone will I suffer
This grief never to leave me.

Nursing me by your own breast
O Mother blest, you raised me

But then Death came so cruelly
Suddenly I'm without you.

. . .

O night, how long and how deep!
Before I'd sleep, you'd hold me tight
Mother, you'd sing through the night
Lest I, in fright, wake and cry

Mother, I wail for your grace
Never again your face will I see
Alone, I burn in agony
What misery, day after day

It's a song that reminds us: we are never alone in our howling grief. These wails
are sacred: our love keen and keening.

As chaplain residents, we always have the option of paging our supervisors for
support. That long, long evening in the ICU, not once does the thought of
asking for help ever cross my mind.

Finally, the family's priest glides in with his vestments and scepter, quiet as a
spring breeze. A stately gentleman, beard graying, the ivory of his bejeweled
cross bright against black robes. Bible and iPhone in hand, he goes to the head
of the bed and begins a liturgy, most of it in Tigre and Geʿez. He makes no
attempt to gather the grieving, just intones on and on, ten minutes, twenty
minutes, thirty minutes. He croons to the woman as if singing her to heaven.
He sheds tears over her bloodstained face.

It is an hour past midnight when he begins to speak extemporaneously. A
family member alerts the priest to my presence. He notices me for the first time,
a Chinese face among a sea of Eritrean ones, and grins. "God bless you!"

Instinctively, I join my palms and bow my head. "Thank you for coming, for
the honor of listening to the beautiful prayers and songs."

His eyes twinkle. "There is life, and there is death, is there not?"

"Death is not an emergency," our supervisors remind us.

The chaplain's role is the opposite of fitting in. While others rush to meet quotas, we pause to make space. What the medical system sees as failure—dying, death—we understand as ineluctable and sacred. When others flee the room, we enter.

Death is not an emergency. Grief is not an emergency. I know this from my supervisors, from the sutras, from Buddhist rituals of mourning that are not finished in a day.

But there is something I forgot that day. None of us are untouched by death. None of us are immune to grief. The deaths and griefs of this world are interconnected. If you were to paint a tableau of that evening, I would be there too, tears threatening to spill over.

·

After meeting the Eritrean priest, I barely sleep a wink. At 9 a.m., I pass the on-call pager to a fellow resident and resolve to make it through the end of the next eight hours.

I don't even make it to lunchtime. My supervisor takes one look at me and tells me to go home.

·

"Chaplains need chaplains too," our supervisors remind us. How easy it is for us caregivers to forget that we too must open ourselves to receiving care.

If I were to set this message to song, I would beseech Indra to descend from Trayastrimsa heaven and regale us as he once did Prince Siddhartha, playing the triple-stringed lute to demonstrate the wisdom of the Middle Way. As the Cambodian Dharma song tradition tells it:

> At first he tuned one string too taut
> and soon that cord snapped in twain.
> Another string, too lax, lacked a crisp twang,
> so he tightened the slack to retune it again.
>
> The moderate way, not too tight or too loose,
> made all fall silent, listening to the strains.
> Strung together in melodies extended or brief,
> the lute sounded sweet in honed harmony.

Once Indra had completely vanished away,
the prince reflected on his realization:
"To inflict austerities misses the mark,
for I've yet to taste the true Dharma.

"Toils and trials cannot defeat conceit.
The crooked path leads only to diversion.
Just like the lute string Indra overstretched,
exertion without ease cannot be endured."[2]

●

Even the chaplaincy visits that sunder us can, upon further reflection, still
us with their insights. The gift of that chaotic evening, the aftermath of that
stormy night, is a blessing for chaplains and other caregivers past, present, and
future:

May our exertions always be companioned by ease

May the merit of our deeds sing to the highest heavens

May we know the taste of true Dharma

Portions of this chapter appear in one long listening: a memoir of grief, friendship, and spiritual care *by Chenxing Han (North Atlantic Books, 2023).*

20

A PLAYFUL DHARMA

Connecting to Our Bodies, Connecting to One Another

Alex Baskin

I.

You don't have to be a dancer to do a one-hand dance. Just take a deep breath and float your fingers up (really, you can do this with me now). Let your hand move around smoothly in any direction you like. Start slowly and then allow the smooth movements to build speed. As your hand flies, switch from smooth motion to jerky. The jerky movements come fast at first; after some time you can move your hand jerky but slowly. Then stop and hold your hand in a shape. Take a breath and feel how that shape feels to you. Now make a really weird shape with your hand. Now make a shape that signifies beauty to you. Now bring your hand to a point of contact with your body. Now move your hand as far from the rest of you as possible. Take another breath and do any combination of these instructions, in any order that feels good to you. This is one way to play.

InterPlay was started by arts educators and "dancing ministers" in Oakland, California, during the 1980s. InterPlay uses creativity to unlock the wisdom of the body. Activities include movement, stillness, voice, sound, breath, and storytelling. It's a bit hard to describe; you learn it best by doing it. I scooted into my first InterPlay group one September with some other Buddhist Harvard Divinity

School (HDS) students. More recently, I worked on an HDS-funded project exploring the connections between Buddhist practice and InterPlay. I read into the literature on play as theology and as pedagogy. I spoke with InterPlay leaders who emphasize the modality's spiritual components and to Buddhist teachers who center embodiment. I attended InterPlay groups and workshops, beamed onto my computer from all over via Zoom video conferencing. A veteran Inter-Play leader coached me on how to guide some basic forms and I started leading online workshops: for teens in mindfulness programs, for young adults in my local meditation community, and for my fellow HDS students.

I am writing this in the year 2020—it's a fraught moment in history. We watched aghast as death claimed innocent lives through an invisible virus and through the centuries-long tentacles of systemic racism. Are times like that really a time for play?

When I talk about playing, I am not thinking of frivolity and I'm definitely not referring to escape. I am speaking about ways of playing that get in touch with reality by experiencing it anew. Consider this painful parallel between the coronavirus pandemic and white supremacy: Both disconnect us from our personal bodies and from the group-body. Remote learning and working meant that many of us stared at screens more than ever, often neglecting how physically tight we became in the process. Plus, our bodies freak many of us out; they remind us of our mortality, which a virus can underline with red marker. Physical-distancing guidelines promote social isolation, leaving us disconnected from one another.

For many, the pandemic meant little experience of hugging a friend. Thus, the era of the coronavirus dissociated us from our bodies and from our neighbors. Systemic racism prompts a corresponding problem. Based on our social-power location, white supremacy leaves us disembodied either through a false—though internalized—sense of superiority or through the pervasive trauma of the threat of violence. The rigid hierarchies of white supremacy control bodies—how bodies can look, what behavior is acceptable, and where bodies can place themselves. (Resmaa Menakem uses the term "white-body supremacy" to emphasize this aspect.)

The construct of race creates a wound in the collective group-body, leaving us separate, segregated, and afraid of one another. These two pandemics (coronavirus and racism) should not be equated as entirely the same. Yet both generate dynamics in which we face difficulties embracing our own bodies and embracing one another. Ideas will not save us. Thinking really hard will not get us out of any of these crises. We need practices that connect us to our bodies and to one another.

Playing allows us to become aware of the body. Buddhist teachings proclaim that the sustained practice of *sati* leads to liberation from suffering. This word from Pāli (the language of early Buddhist texts) is often translated as "mind-fulness," though it has no etymological relationship to the word "mind." *Sati* is derived from the term for "memory"—we remember to maintain awareness of what we do as we do it. "Bodyfulness" is as good a translation. The Buddha talked about bringing sati to all activities: standing, walking, eating, getting dressed, and going to the bathroom. Silent, still-bodied meditation is just one way to train in sati. It is not the whole path to liberation, and it does not work best for everyone. Many of us need to wiggle more. When I get up from my meditation cushion, from a laptop screen, or from a book (as I invite you to do for a moment right now) and shake, or stretch, or squirm for several seconds, I remember what it feels like to be a human body (seriously, please, look away from this and move for a brief moment).

Not only does playing develop our body awareness, but it also connects us to others. Buddhist traditions maintain that Sangha, a Pāli term often translated as "community," is one of the only sources of reliable refuge in our chaotic world. We do not just need really good self-care. We need one another. When we create something like a hand-dance with others, taking turns, riffing off the movement we just witnessed, we become attuned to those we are playing with. We build community, not as an abstract notion, but as a somatic relationship.

Even over Zoom, InterPlayers report feeling less isolated after these activities. Perhaps it seems naive to propose play as a response to racism. Of course, embodied practices need to happen alongside radical political restructuring. Yet creative expression in communities that are affirming and inclusive ought to be a part of the process of healing our history of disconnection and violence. This is a way to use relationality as a refuge for charting a path toward liberation from suffering.

II.

I first became curious about theorizing connections between Buddhism and play when I read Courtney Goto's writing on Christian theology and play. She proposes that playing helps us understand revelatory experiencing and God's new creation. This led me to wonder how an investigation like Goto's would proceed if applied to Buddhist theology. I grew excited about the relevance of play to sati and Sangha and other Buddhist concepts as well. Yet, part of the brilliance of InterPlay is its nondidactic pedagogy—InterPlay is proud to declare its "sneaky-deep" methodology. We just play. Leaders don't tell participants what kind of experience they are supposed to have. Yet when we stop and report how one InterPlay form or another is landing in our bodies (this "noticing" being a key ingredient in InterPlay's magic), similar reactions inevitably emerge. We hear that InterPlayers feel more connected to the body, more connected to one another, more aware, lighter, more resilient. Of course, it is not all jolly and merry—through play we encounter our woundedness too. But importantly, these embodied creative tools themselves foster healing.

A huge learning in my project emerged when I realized that I didn't have to make the case that Buddhism and play have something to offer each other. Rather than impress anyone with my nifty theorizing, I could just guide some meditation practices, juxtapose them with InterPlay forms, and allow those present to arrive at their own conclusions.

When I led workshops, the participants did not disappoint. One person reflected that she noticed the overlapping terrain of movement and silent meditation—both tap into something beyond language, something in our phenomenological world that we cannot put into words. Someone in the workshop used a storytelling form to voice his frustrations about and wishes for our local meditation community, which was thus cathartic and fostered bonding. So many "noticings" (those self-reports in the midst of InterPlay practice) referenced joy—a canonical Buddhist value that was described by the Buddha as a component of deep meditation states, a step in the awakening process, and a foundational heart-meditation practice.

III.

What does this have to do with crisis care, the theme of the present volume? For one, play can support those who care for others. We know that caregivers shoulder a heavy burden and need ways to rest and rejuvenate. Joyful, embodied practices can serve that purpose. Another possible connection: Embodied creativity represents spiritual care in its own right. Those in crisis benefit from connecting to their bodies and to others, which playfulness offers. One close-knit InterPlay group devoted sessions over a nine-month period to a member of the cohort who was dying of cancer. She was able to physically act out her emotions—moving with and through them—tell stories, sing, and joke about the pain she was enduring. When I heard about that group, I recognized it as a form of spiritual care.

But it is not just that playfulness can serve as self-care and as spiritual care. It blurs lines too, disrupting any neat division between caring for ourselves and caring for others. In one InterPlay form, a dyad alternates following and leading. The first person holds up, let's say, a palm and the follower mirrors by holding up a palm as well. The leader maybe curls each finger in, turning the palm into a fist. The other person copies that. The fist swings up and out toward the ceiling; again the action is reflected. Before long, the follower and leader switch roles. The new leader offers gestures and movements for the new follower to mimic. But then something really exciting happens. In the third phase, after each member of the pair has been the official leader, the roles are dropped altogether. With no clear leader, the dyad moves freely, trying their best to continue mirroring each other. Through micro-acts of leading and following, both surprise each other with their ability to stay more-or-less in sync. It's fuzzy: Am I leading or am I following? Am I giving care or am I receiving it?

This blur is fortunate because all of us suffer and all of us care for those who are suffering. In InterPlay, we point out that because stress is physical, grace (the opposite of stress) is too. We experience grace in the body, and we can cultivate grace—for ourselves and for others. It is not about pretending to feel good when we don't. But we can engage in active practices that foster a feeling. Play is like cultivating heart-qualities, such as *mettā* (loving-kindness) or compassion. We may not be feeling loving-kindness toward all living beings, but engaging in the repetition of mettā phrases can often prompt the feeling to arise (a common Buddhist practice, repeating: "May I be happy, safe, and at ease / May all beings be happy, safe, and at ease"). We can have joy in our bodies through playful movement. We imagine what the physicality of grace is like (the way we feel in the forest, or under comfy blankets, or hugging a grandparent) and we actively recreate it. We cultivate grace in the body—a vital practice for caregivers and care seekers.

IV.

I have been sensing the ripple effects of these sneaky-deep practices in my body and heart. I feel light, bouncy, joyful, and when I am feeling crunchy, tense, or anxious, I have ways to play and discharge that energy too. My Buddhist practice, which has been a part of my life for a while, has been reinvigorated through embodied movement and the ethos of play. I feel more awake and more liberated. By playing as a spiritual endeavor, I touch deeply into Dharma—encapsulating the term from Sanskrit (the language of many late Buddhist texts), which denotes spiritual-religious practice as well as referring to reality itself. Hence, my Dharma is a playful one.

Take a deep breath and let it out with an audible sigh. Try that a couple of times. Let your exhales get goofy. Roar like a lion. Whisper something sweet and romantic to yourself. Don't take my word for it—see for yourself: How does that feel in your body?

I would like to express my appreciation to Roselyn Bell and C. C. King for their help in editing this chapter.

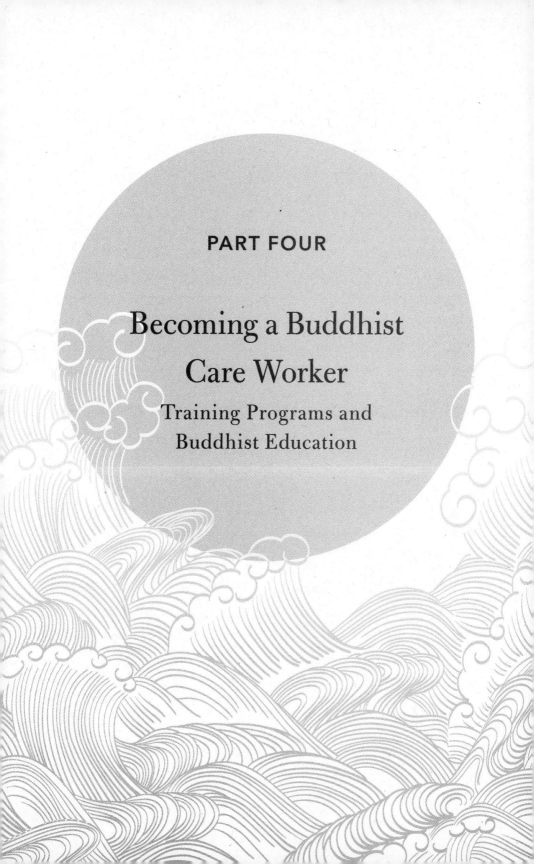

PART FOUR

Becoming a Buddhist Care Worker

Training Programs and Buddhist Education

21

THE HEART
CONSULTATION ROOM

Post-Disaster Care and Adapting
Chaplaincy in Japan

Taniyama Yōzō, PhD

S hortly after the devastating Triple Disaster of 2011, we established the Heart Consultation Room in Sendai, the largest city near the earthquake epicenter, where volunteers from various religious traditions tried to help meet the emotional and spiritual needs of people in the area. The Heart Consultation Room was strictly nondenominational. Even if many volunteers were Buddhist, it transcended any religious boundaries. People from different faiths worked together to care for survivors, hold memorials for victims, and also to care for distressed caregivers themselves.

Just four days after the disaster, a Jōdo Buddhist priest who was the general secretary of the Sendai Buddhist Association, Nakamura Mizuki, advocated for volunteer sutra readers at funeral homes. Because of the vast damage during the disaster, it necessitated large numbers of the population to move away from their hometown areas to other parts of their prefecture and even into other regions of Japan. Being forced into that position on such short notice is incredibly difficult for any individual or family, but it also has important implications for grief care and Japanese Buddhist beliefs and traditions. It raises questions about how the Buddhist organizations can properly support those people. How are they able to do a funeral or memorial for their loved ones or continue their ancestor veneration?

In Japan, even most families who have only remote connections to Buddhism in their daily lives still prefer Buddhist memorials. There are common beliefs—especially in northern Japan where the tsunami hit—that souls may not properly advance toward Buddhahood like they otherwise would without a proper memorial and sutra chanting. For many Japanese, Buddhist altars in people's homes and memorial tablets of ancestors who passed away are more than just precious objects. People usually act as if those objects contain the presence of those who passed away. These altars and tablets represent the bond that connects the living and the dead. They are often treated as family members themselves in value and importance. So, in Japan, they also represent a critical part of the grief care. Caregivers have to bear in mind that to lose those objects and be so far away from where they were lost can cause deep pain in itself. Memorial services also bear a vital role in grief care. A decent funeral and memorial service can help calm an already stressed and traumatized family. In so doing, memorials can also provide great relief to family members struggling with their grief. The tsunami in particular took so many lives during the tragedy and destroyed so many buildings that there was an immense shortage of the necessary places and people to lead religious services that people were demanding.

One of the critical figures in helping to set up post-disaster care activities was Okabe Takeshi (1950–2012). Okabe was one of the pioneers of palliative care in Japan, founding a clinic in Sendai that helped organize in-home care for thousands of patients. He also helped start a local research and discussion group on dying. By 2010, however, Okabe discovered he too had cancer and would have to consider his own dying process. Although he was told that he only had ten months to live, Okabe lived through the 2011 disaster that came around that time. A respected nurse from his clinic's staff, however, was a victim, and there was immense grief felt by the entire staff. Through the calming feeling Okabe and the staff finally felt as Buddhist priests chanted sutras during the memorial service, Okabe viscerally felt the power that rituals can have in the grieving process. Prior to this, Okabe harbored doubts about chaplaincy and the role of religion in palliative care. But this experience led him to accept it on a far deeper level and to volunteer alongside Buddhist priests in their post-disaster care. He found that, for grieving families of disaster victims, rather than talking to doctors, nurses, or psychologists, it was the presence of those with religious authority who had the deepest impact.

By cooperating with other religious groups, volunteers were able to ensure that the memorial services would not favor any specific religious group. Thus, they negotiated with the local city government to allow them the use of a two-floor building to conduct various forms of care for survivors within and around the community. Soon after it opened, this "Heart Consultation Room" was conducting memorials almost unceasingly every day. While clergy from different religions, including a wide variety of Buddhist sects, led these services on the first floor, the second floor was used for other forms of care.

The government-negotiated facility was only available for two months after the disaster, but people's needs were far from over. Luckily, Tohoku University, a renowned university in the region, was able not only to house the memorials during subsequent months, but also to add additional care-related activities. This is also when I began volunteering with the Heart Consultation Room. One service was a café setting with volunteers available not only to serve drinks and snacks, but also to listen to those who needed to talk, share their stories of the tragedy, and have the presence of another by their side (this mobile café is discussed in chapter 6, "Café de Monk"). The Heart Consultation Room also operated a call center through which those who couldn't come in person could talk to clergy about their problems. Other activities included a radio station that broadcast "messages from the heart" to provide calming and uplifting stories and messages.

One issue, however, is that chaplaincy and religious involvement within public forms of care in Japan are very new within modern society. Even if Buddhism was historically involved in many forms of medical and spiritual care for many centuries, Buddhism's role began to fade with modernization. Then, after World War II, the separation of religion and state was far stricter than in most Western nations. Chaplains in a public hospital, for example, cannot freely perform a religious ceremony even if requested by the patient. This leads us to make clearer distinctions in Japan between "religious care" and "spiritual care." Describing these two forms of care, Kubotera Toshiyuki states, "Both are types of care that deal with a soul-level of pain that is deeper than psychological pain. They both deal with transcendent issues beyond what the normal eye can see. Where they differ is the approach that one takes to address the needs of the care recipient."[1]

One difference is that those offering religious care provide specific "answers" to questions people look to hear from their own particular religious traditions. It's the relationship between a believer and an ordained expert of a tradition. But with spiritual care, we assume that the world view, values, and beliefs may not be the same between the caregiver and care recipient. Rather than providing answers, they help work together with the care recipient to explore the questions and come to certain self-realizations. Especially during times of crisis, both types of care can provide essential support.

What is critical, though, is for clergy to be aware of these two different frames of care so that when they are serving someone during a time of crisis, they are truly supporting the individuals' needs. This can be particularly difficult in public settings in Japan. Chaplains who belong to one particular religion or sect of Buddhism must know about the rituals of other sects. I am a priest in the Ōtani branch of Jōdo Shinshū Buddhism. But when I began caring for survivors of the 2011 disaster, I learned the basics for chanting in several other Buddhist traditions: Sōtō Zen, Jōdo, Nichiren, and Shingon. We had to meet the needs of survivors who came from many varying traditions.

One important aspect of care was grief care, and in this post-disaster context, the meaning of grief care took on a particularly broad range of human reactions. Survivors of the earthquake and tsunami not only lost family, they grieved for many other parts of their lives that were literally swept away. Homes were gone. Family heirlooms and other precious objects were gone. Many people from along the coast had to settle in new areas of the country, starting their lives from scratch. In some cases, there was not even a village to return to, as nearly everything from the person's hometown was gone. Jobs and other nonmaterial aspects of life constituted another aspect of loss and grief. Pile all of these on top of one another and you can imagine how deep the sadness and grief were for many of these people to deal with.

When I was helping at the Heart Consultation Room, Buddhist volunteers were striving for a system to coordinate their grief care with medical care. Due to my previous experience as a hospice chaplain at Japan's first Buddhist hospice, I had more experience working with the medical community than most volunteers and was able to garner their trust. It was thus easier for me to work as an intermediary between these fields and help reorganize the cooperative efforts of the Heart Consultation Room. By the time the facility moved to Tohoku University, we were also able to add chaplain training to the list of activities. As much as the volunteers from Buddhist traditions and other religions wanted to help, it was difficult for someone with no experience in disaster care to know how to listen to or speak with survivors. We also recognized a longer-term need for people to have this training. The grief experienced by disaster survivors is deep and multilayered. By increasing the people trained in spiritual care, we can have a much greater capacity to attend to all the needs of the people.

Okabe Takeshi wanted to deepen his cooperation with religious professionals and was instrumental in helping to initiate this training. Okabe dedicated the final year of his life to helping create better cooperation between the religious and medical fields and helping to establish interfaith chaplaincy in Japan. He even helped train one Zen priest in chaplaincy by using himself as a practice patient, training another through his own dying experience. The founder of the listening café, Kaneta Taiō (the subject of chapter 6), also helped lead the early stages of this training.

Another important step is actually introducing spiritual care to the Japanese people. Most Japanese are still unfamiliar with chaplaincy and, in modern Japan, it is very strange to see Buddhist priests in certain settings, like a hospital or hospice. Because Japanese people associate Buddhist priests with funerals and times of death, it can even be scary for a sick person to encounter a priest while still alive. Priests in Japan are also far more accustomed to preaching to parishioners and speaking from their own sectarian perspectives than listening to a patient and meeting the spiritual needs of those from a different tradition. Yet, on the other hand, these priests are experienced in talking about death and dying, and there are a deep history and tradition with elements of grief care in Buddhism. They also have experience in the various forms of religious care that can be helpful and calming in the dying process. Therefore, Buddhist priests already have many of the tools necessary to help them become good chaplains with proper training. We thought that these chaplaincy skills could be useful not only in those cases of disaster care, but throughout hospitals, hospices, and other places of more regular need in Japan.

Regarding the issue of the lack of familiarity with chaplaincy in Japan, Dr. Okabe thought it might be best to create a new Japanese word to help people understand the role. Rather than the adapted word *chapuren,* which replicates the English sound of the word, Okabe preferred to use *kanji* characters that represented a combination of the words for "clinical," "religious," and "teacher or expert." When this new word, 臨床宗教師 *(rinshōshūkyōshi),* was seen by the average Japanese person, they could at least have a general idea regarding the person's role by seeing the characters. Introducing a new field and role into a society is not a short process, but gratefully, rinshōshūkyōshi and the training for them have spread quite amply in the time since then. We created a certifying organization to recognize those who complete the training, the Society for Interfaith Chaplaincy in Japan. Besides Tohoku University, as of 2022 there are eight other universities and organizations registered to train rinshōshūkyōshi, and we have certified over two hundred chaplains in total. Hopefully this field will continue to grow so that we may better meet the needs of not only disaster victims, but many others' spiritual needs as time goes on.

Translated by Nathan Jishin Michon.

22

AGING IN CHINA AND THE LIFE CARE PROGRAM OF SHANGHAI JADE BUDDHA TEMPLE

Wang Fengshuo

Introduction

Death for Chinese people is a taboo, yet it is one of the four cardinal life events—birth, aging, illness, and death—that everyone will have to face. While China has prenatal classes to prepare for the birth of a baby, there are no pre-death classes to prepare for a family member's passing, let alone one's own death. In 2000, China's population aged sixty-five and older accounted for 7 percent of the total population, which means that China entered the category of an "aging society." Shanghai is the first city to enter this designation, and it is also the city with the highest degree of aging. According to the latest data, in 2009 the number of elderly people aged sixty and older in Shanghai was 5.2 million, accounting for 35.2 percent of all registered urban residents. Confronting the aging problem in China, Shanghai Jade Buddha Temple established the Life Education College to open courses on thanatology, hospice care, and more. As an urban temple in central Shanghai, Jade Buddha Temple is a case study to see how a Buddhist temple in a large city adapts to new social changes.

This chapter uses Jade Buddha Temple as an example to illustrate how Chinese Buddhism is involved in Chinese social issues, and especially the aging crisis that Shanghai and the nation as a whole continues to face. The first part of this chapter provides a short introduction to the history of hospice care in

China, with a focus on the current development of hospice care in Shanghai. The second part takes Shanghai Jade Buddha Temple as an example to describe its life care program. The third part discusses how the life care program relates to the sinicization of religion in China.

Hospice Care in Shanghai

According to the World Health Organization, the aim of hospice care is to improve the quality of life of those with terminal illness until the end of their life. Hospice care in China officially began in 1987 with the founding of Beijing Songtang Care Hospital.

Shanghai, China's most aged city, has since become a leading city for hospice care. In 1988, the first hospice care ward opened in Nanhui County Elderly Care Hospital, and six years later, the first research center for the study of hospice care was established in Shanghai Linfen Hospital. Although hospice care became known to Shanghai residents in the late 1980s, people seldom chose hospice care at the end of their lives.

In 2012, Shanghai's hospice care saw a turning point. That year, Qin Ling, a high school Chinese teacher, wrote a letter to the secretary of the municipal party committee, Yu Zhengsheng. Qin Ling's father suffered from incurable lung cancer, and there was no hospital willing to accept him. This letter quickly attracted the attention of Yu. He replied that "We will try our best to help you." The same year, the Shanghai government began the construction of community hospice care facilities. From then through 2020, all 246 community health service centers in Shanghai launched hospice care service. Among them, 217 community health centers rely on family beds to provide home hospice care service, 106 centers provide hospice care ward service, and 98 centers offer both services. A total of 8,000 professionals are engaged in hospice care service. From September 2019 to August 2020, about 11,600 patients chose hospice care.[1]

Unlike Western countries, Shanghai's hospice care has strong government guidance. Because of China's policy that religious activities can only be conducted in religious areas, monks, nuns, and priests are not allowed to provide hospice care service at hospitals. Therefore, religious communities' involvement in hospice care in China becomes a challenging issue.

Life Education and Jade Buddha Temple

The Life Care Project

The origin of Jade Buddha Temple can be traced back to the Guangxu Period of the Qing Dynasty. In 1882, Master Hui Gen took a pilgrimage to India. During his journey back to China, he passed through Burma and brought back five jade Buddha statues. Two statues were left in Shanghai, and a hut built to consecrate the two jade Buddha statues developed into the Jade Buddha Temple.

Over Jade Buddha Temple's history of nearly a century and a half, the way of promoting Buddhism has changed from traditional Dharma transmission at the temple to a modern humanistic Buddhist way of acting compassionately in this world. One clear consequence has been changes in Buddhist forms of charity.

From the late 1980s, Jade Buddha Temple began to carry out charitable activities in the traditional way of donation. After stepping into the twenty-first century, members of Jade Buddha Temple gradually found that the mere donation of money was not the best way to help people. A more professional organization was needed.

In February 2015, Jade Buddha Temple established Shanghai's first non-public fund for a foundation for culture and education with a registered capital of about $460,000. Known as Juequn Culture and Education Foundation, it marked a major shift in the temple's economic and social engagement. From this time on, the operation of Buddhist charity in the way of a foundation has substituted for the traditional way of donation.

The foundation began by launching projects such as Loving Library, Chinese Traditional Education for Children, and others. But these projects could also be carried out by other organizations. Foundation members began to wonder if there was a better project to embody a specifically Buddhist vision. In 2018, the Juequn foundation concluded that its efforts would be better focused on life care. With the expectation to build a theoretical system of Buddhist thanatology and guide the public to have a new understanding of life, the foundation officially launched the life care project. As a newcomer into the field, the foundation started by cooperating with both local hospital medical staff and a university scholar to work jointly on the project. During the following two years, it established cooperative relationships with seventy-six community health centers and organized an international conference titled "Buddhist Approaches to Hospice Care and Life Education." At this conference, there were more than twenty scholars from the United States, Sri Lanka, Britain, Japan, Singapore, Thailand, and other countries participating and discussing life care.

As the program moved forward, the coming of the COVID-19 pandemic resulted in a stagnation of program development. After the outbreak of the crisis, as a safety precaution none of the hospitals or community service centers allowed volunteers to enter. Therefore, all of the face-to-face hospice care volunteer service by Shanghai's nongovernment organizations halted. The volunteers had more time but fewer opportunities to help. To respond to the crisis, several life care organizations began to use iPads and smartphones to accompany patients online, but the accompaniment time was shortened to half an hour. The social need for providing hospice care service to hospitals is now shifting to the need for volunteers to improve their skills. This influenced the program at Jade Buddha Temple to change its emphasis from service to education.

From Project to College

The pandemic impacted many fields, and religious practice is no exception. Starting from the 2020 Chinese New Year, Jade Buddha Temple was closed for more than half a year, and the main task of the temple transitioned to the fight against COVID-19. During this period, the temple realized that people not only suffer physically but also mentally and spiritually. There is no course in Chinese school telling children how to face illness and death. When these children grow up, they lack the necessary knowledge and skills to handle negative emotions and feelings. The consequences become particularly obvious during a widespread crisis. Therefore, a more systematic education in life care was desperately needed in China.

This realization transformed the life care program from separate projects into a systematic education system. After the temple reopened in June, the foundation began to prepare for the establishment of "Life Education College" and held an opening ceremony on October 17, 2020.

To provide life care service for people of all ages, the college planned to open courses in the following four fields: (1) hospice care, (2) mental health of children and youth, (3) mindfulness-based stress reduction for people living in big cities, and (4) elderly care. Because the foundation has accumulated many experiences in hospice care service, it starts with a preliminary-level teacher-training program in hospice care.

The preliminary-level teacher-training program has two courses. In the first class, after the temple posted a notification about the teacher-training program, 193 people applied to take part, and forty-four participants were selected after exams and interviews. Due to the success of the first class, the second class enrolled sixty-six students, and some students even came from other cities. They spent three weekends studying life philosophy, psychology, and caring skills with seventeen medical and psychological experts. The temple covers all the cost of training, but students have to pledge to do at least one hundred hours of volunteer work within two years after graduation. These students' ages ranged from twenty to sixty-two, and a significant number of them are Buddhists.

The intermediate-level and advanced-level classes of the teacher-training program in hospice care were held in 2021. Those students who successfully passed the preliminary-level class exams were entitled to attend the subsequent classes. After completing the whole training, these trained students are awarded a Hospice Care Giver Certificate and have an opportunity to do service at hospitals or spread life care knowledge in community centers and nursing homes. These hospitals, nursing homes, and community centers have close cooperative relationships with the temple.

Apart from opening courses, Juequn Life Education College also aims to establish its own broader curriculum of life care education. The courses in Buddhist thanatology, Eastern and Western philosophy in life care, educational theory, and so on, are still in the developmental process as of this writing. Hopefully in the future, a more comprehensive Buddhist chaplaincy education will appear in China.

The temple also hopes that in the future, there will be three branches in the college: a registrar's office responsible for course arrangement, a research center responsible for research on Buddhist chaplaincy and thanatology, and a project management department responsible for connecting volunteers and community. The temple has a vision that in the future, Chinese Buddhist temples will have the capability to run their own nursing homes.

Life Care and Sinicization

When Buddhism entered China during the Han Dynasty, it went through a process of sinicization by integrating with Chinese culture. This process has accelerated particularly after 2016, when President Xi Jinping proposed adhering to the sinicization of religions and proactively guiding religions to adapt to socialist society. The life care program of Jade Buddha Temple is a window for us to glimpse the sinicization of Chinese Buddhism in contemporary China.

To adapt to the paradigm of socialist society as prescribed by the government, Life Education College aims to not merely spread Buddhism but to administer to aspects of suffering within the everyday lives of people in the environs of Shanghai. The courses directly related to Buddhism only occupy a small portion of the whole program. Most coursework is centered in the fields of psychology, philosophy, and social work. Students acquire a general understanding of Buddhist philosophy and thus know how to communicate with patients in the Buddhist faith. Therefore, the courses are more service-centered than Buddhism-centered. The state religious policy that monastics cannot enter hospitals to provide service also affects the course design of the college, meaning that it relies on lay teaching staff from hospitals and universities. Therefore, neither teacher nor students within the program are monastics.

Conclusion

In comparison to chaplaincy and care education in Western countries, Chinese Buddhist chaplaincy lags behind. There are no systematic courses offering spiritual care and multifaith knowledge to those in need. To comply with religious policies, monks and nuns are not currently allowed to be trained as professional chaplains, but it is still possible to have lay Buddhists and volunteers participate in service. How Chinese temples develop a systematic Buddhist chaplaincy adaptable to Chinese society is still an issue the Jade Buddha Temple and other Chinese Buddhists must continue to explore and develop.

The life care program of Jade Buddha Temple is at least one step in that direction. The program was initiated with the backdrop of the sinicization of religion in aging China. To respond to the aging crisis in China, Jade Buddha Temple established Life Education College to open teacher-training courses for hospice care in 2020. Although the college is exploring a sinicized way of implementing Buddhist chaplaincy, the shortage of systematic education in life care makes it obvious that there is still a long way to go for Chinese Buddhist Chaplaincy and caregiving to develop in the future.

23

THE PATH TO BUDDHIST CHAPLAINCY IN THE UNITED STATES

Academic Education, Religious Endorsement, Professional Board Certification

Jitsujo T. Gauthier, PhD; Daijaku Judith Kinst, PhD; Leigh Miller, PhD; Elaine Yuen, PhD

Introduction

Many people interested in the application of Buddhist or contemplative religious practices to alleviate the suffering of other people are discovering chaplaincy or spiritual care as a professional calling. Cultivating a Buddhist practice that strengthens inner qualities and resources—such as compassion, insight into interdependence, and reduced reification of "self"—builds capacity for offering presence and fearlessness in the face of others' sufferings. These, it turns out, are vital qualifications for spiritual care providers. As the profession and practitioners both begin to recognize a mutual good fit, it's worthwhile to explore the emergence of Buddhist chaplaincy, the contributions Buddhist teachings and practices can make to chaplaincy, the training that is required and available for people wishing to pursue this path of Right Livelihood, and the challenges that exist in the development and professionalization of chaplains from a minority religion in the United States.

Buddhist chaplaincy emerged as a form of engaged and humanistic Buddhism into the larger field of chaplaincy within the Judeo-Christian context of the United States. During the early 1900s, professional chaplaincy in the United States developed standards of education, clinical training, spiritual formation, ethical competencies, and certification. Recently a think tank called the Chaplaincy Innovation Lab was created through Brandeis University, bringing together chaplains, educators, researchers, and clinical supervisors from a range of settings and traditions to spark "practical innovations that enable chaplains to nurture the spirits of those they serve and reduce human suffering."[1] While Buddhist chaplaincy is relatively young, it nonetheless has unique offerings to make to the larger chaplaincy field in terms of contemplative praxis, presence, and reflexivity. The field of Buddhist chaplaincy is beginning to form ethical standards of role, competence, and endorsement, which align with the larger professional field, as well as to consider perspectives within the Buddhist context of history, culture, and tradition. This chapter offers an overview of these developments, particularly for those interested in seeking an academic degree, endorsement, and a career that will align their spiritual values with existing, recognized professional and educational requirements.

The emergence of Buddhist chaplaincy can be contextualized within the growth of Buddhism as a minority religion in the United States, presenting unique needs and opportunities for Buddhist practitioners and Buddhist communities. Many people in general are turning to Buddhist leaders and communities for guidance through self-other understanding, suffering, and emotional-spiritual development. This raises questions about the identification of religious roles and how best to prepare people in various roles to meet these needs: compassionately, skillfully, ethically, and with mature spiritual authority. In part this is shaped by traditions within Buddhist lineages and schools. Additionally, as Buddhist Sanghas are expanding and growing throughout the United States, the kinds of pastoral-spiritual care and counseling skills associated with training for chaplains and clergy in the United States are becoming, for some Buddhist teachers, spiritual leaders, priests, ministers, and senior students, more and more necessary.

In 2014 the Buddhist Ministry Working Group formed through a Buddhist Ministry Initiative conference at Harvard Divinity School.[2] The group, comprising Buddhist chaplaincy educators and Sangha leaders, has been working together to create and support a comprehensive collaboration within a mutually supportive network of Buddhist educational institutions involved in the development of students and the field of Buddhist ministry. The intention of this group is to cultivate the specific field of Buddhist chaplaincy, as well as the broader field of Buddhist ministry, to include leadership training and community service.

A lack of awareness and clarity around the current field of Buddhist chaplaincy and ministry can confuse professional boundaries, dissemination of knowledge, and ethical standards. In order for future Buddhist chaplains to thrive in healthy ways, the standards of practice, roles, and competencies need to be clarified. Buddhist Chaplaincy development (formation) is both an acquisition of skills and knowledge and a cultivation of inner qualities resulting in personal ripening. Professional certification as a chaplain in the United States follows three main criteria: (1) educational, (2) clinical, and (3) community endorsement. Once these criteria are met, a chaplain candidate may apply for professional certification. Given the newness around Buddhist chaplaincy education and endorsement in particular, there has been some flexibility for creating equivalencies in these areas; however, this may become the exception moving forward. The most common field of chaplaincy employment in the United States is within health care. Outside health care, standards for professional employment can differ, and outside the military, standards are generally less strict and can lack requirements for professional certification. However, most other chaplains still follow much of the same training as health-care chaplains. That being the standard, this chapter will follow those requirements. The following sections attempt to outline processes of training, religious education, endorsement, and certification for those interested in becoming a Buddhist chaplain. The authors aim to note the highest standards necessary in order to meet care recipients in ways that are mutually beneficial, ethically sound, and from the heart.

Chaplaincy Professional Certification Requirements for Buddhist Chaplains

There are four requirements for the highest standard of professional chaplaincy in the United States. Buddhist chaplains with professional certification would complete:

1. Educational training: A 72-unit accredited graduate degree in Buddhist chaplaincy or the equivalent as determined by the Association of Professional Chaplains. A degree may be a Master of Divinity (MDiv) or Master of Arts (MA).

2. Clinical training: 4 units (one year total) of clinical training from approved clinical pastoral education (CPE) chaplaincy internship-residency programs.

3. Endorsement: Received from the Buddhist community within which the chaplain candidate identifies and practices.

4. Board certification: Received from the Association of Professional Chaplains (APC), which requires additional employment as a chaplain and a certification review process.

Education Requirements

This section will focus on discussion of the academic religious or "theological" education required. Students interested in becoming a Buddhist chaplain often enroll in an accredited college or university to complete the required seventy-two-unit graduate degree and earn a Master of Divinity (MDiv) or Master of Arts (MA) in Buddhist chaplaincy. An accredited college, university, or educational institute or organization is authorized to confer academic degrees by a national organization (such as the Association of Theological Schools), or a regional organization that is recognized by the national Council for Higher Education Accreditation (such as the Western Association for Schools and Colleges). Some states also have accrediting bodies (for example, the Higher Educational Coordinating Commission of Oregon), which oversees and enforces educational standards. Other states, for example California, do not have such state accrediting bodies. Accredited Buddhist chaplaincy educational programs are visited and reviewed by the accrediting body to ensure that their curricula, faculty, administration, and other elements align with national, regional, or state educational requirements and academic standards. Accreditation from national or regional accrediting bodies, authorized by the U.S. Department of Education, serves as the imprimatur of a degree program's validity, ensuring it will be recognized nationally and internationally by other schools and employers as a credential.

The Association of Professional Chaplains requires that applicants for APC board certification have either an accredited seventy-two-unit graduate theological degree or successfully demonstrate comparable religious educational training through the APC's Theological Educational Equivalency process. Prior to the advent of accredited Buddhist chaplaincy graduate programs, this was a particularly important way that Buddhists received recognition for training in Buddhist temples, monasteries, or settings other than accredited universities. This continues to be a viable path.

To guide the assessment of the religious and educational training accrued by individual Buddhists while also creating common standards recognizable across diverse Buddhist traditions, the APC in 2006 worked with a Buddhist task force to create a white paper.[3] This white paper has served to assist Buddhist chaplains in developing equivalencies for certification by recognizing their Dharma training, mentorship, meditation retreats, and rituals. This has been helpful, but the Buddhist white paper was formulated before many U.S. Buddhist chaplaincy MA and MDiv programs existed. More recently, pathways for APC recognition of educational training from institutions without federal accreditation have included assessment of that institution's educational program curricula. For instance, the APC assessed the MDiv program at Maitripa College, which holds degree-granting authority in the State of Oregon, and determined that its graduate degrees would be recognized as the theological educational equivalent of accredited degrees, thus eliminating the need for individual candidate applicants to pursue the APC equivalency process on a case-by-case basis. Similarly, the Buddhist Chaplaincy Training Program at Upaya Zen Center in Santa Fe, New Mexico, has been assessed by the APC as the theological educational equivalent of forty-eight graduate credits.

Current Buddhist chaplaincy MDiv and MA program educational standards align with the academic degree requirements of the APC. The APC identifies thirteen essential areas of study that apply to MDiv curricula in any religious tradition. Categories of study include courses in religious history, foundational religious teachings and tenets, sacred texts, ethical frameworks and development, world religions or comparative religions, ethnic and cultural diversity, chaplaincy, spiritual care and counseling, communications skills, spiritual or religious education, professional ethics, spiritual or religious leadership within communities and organizations, and supervised faith-based internships. Religious studies classes teach the philosophy, hermeneutics, texts, and canonical languages of Buddhism. Degree programs may offer coursework that emphasizes some areas more than others according to their university and program mission, values, and philosophies. However, all programs cover all thirteen areas. Degree programs may also vary in philosophy, organization, and how pedagogy reflects the founding Buddhist tradition based on the age of the program, geographic location, and faculty. In addition, students may choose an area of focus that interests them.

All programs aim to support and guide the student in developing a sound basis for their practice of Buddhist chaplaincy. Curricula may include classes on the history, texts, teachings, and practices of Buddhism, the history and theoretical foundations of chaplaincy, spiritual formation, contemplative care and counseling practices, structures of power and privilege, Buddhist ministry, leadership, and pastoral care, interfaith dialogue, and competence in non-Buddhist traditions. Chaplaincy classes are often interdisciplinary and include a range of relevant topics, including communication and counseling skills, healthy boundaries, and power dynamics within professional and personal relationships. Buddhist educational programs weave in non-Buddhist sources and methods of assessment, care, and counseling. Students learn how to build bridges to non-Buddhist faith-based systems and apply Buddhist scriptures to real-life situations. Classes are sometimes also open to Buddhist community leaders outside the degree program.

Internship and Residency Programs

Educational programs also consider clinical standards, which are outlined by the Association of Clinical Pastoral Education (ACPE) when devising curricula. ACPE accredits clinical pastoral education programs where Buddhist chaplains complete internships and residency training to gain hands-on experience.

Most CPE programs throughout the United States are housed in hospital systems, though some hospices have CPE programs, and some CPE programs place chaplain interns and residents in universities, prisons, nonprofit organizations, and temple, church, and community settings. CPE internships are usually one unit, 300 clinical hours plus 100 educational hours, offered part-time or full-time. CPE residencies are usually three or four units over the course of a year and offer modest stipends. Although most Buddhist chaplaincy educational and clinical programs highly value in-person learning, some programs are exploring online or hybrid learning in order to provide distance learning opportunities for a diversity of students.

Endorsement

In addition to education and clinical training requirements, aspiring board certified chaplains (BCC) are required to obtain endorsement from their faith community. The purpose of endorsement is to ensure that the endorsee is educationally, doctrinally, and developmentally qualified to represent their faith community in the specialized setting of chaplaincy. It is an acknowledgment, in the form of a letter from a faith community, that certifies that the endorsee has the knowledge and pastoral ability to represent their tradition and provide spiritual care to others facing sickness, trauma, and death.[4] Endorsement will only be recognized by the APC if it is conferred by a faith-based endorsing body approved by the APC.

The process of APC/Board Certified Chaplain Inc. (BCCI) certification can be challenging for some Buddhists, particularly if they seek educational equivalency. For some, obtaining endorsement can also pose a challenge. There are less than fifty certified Buddhist chaplains in the United States as of 2018, and only around twenty Buddhist communities currently approved by the APC as faith-based endorsing bodies. One reason for this has been that the religious professional role of a "chaplain" has neither been part of Asian traditions nor the formation of Buddhist communities in the West.

More recently, the APC called on a second Buddhist task force comprising individuals from Buddhist chaplaincy MDiv and MA and training programs in the United States. Their task was to create (1) a user-friendly endorsement form for both the endorser (a Buddhist teacher or community) and the endorsee by adapting language from the original Christian endorsement process, and

(2) a structure to ensure that those applying for certification are affiliated with a recognized Buddhist lineage, tradition, or organization. The APC recognizes that for most religious communities, the spiritual maturity of the endorsee is recognized and determined according to the standards articulated within that community. They seek to both uphold professional standards and also to adapt to the unique needs of aspiring Buddhist chaplains.

The resulting new "Faith-based Community Endorsing Body Recognition" application for Buddhists was completed in 2018 and is available on request from the APC. Buddhists seeking board certification are encouraged to take this form to the leadership of their Buddhist communities and develop processes and materials collaboratively. Examples from other recognized Buddhist endorsing communities may offer helpful models.

APC Certification Overview

The APC is considered the primary certifying body because it upholds the highest standards for becoming a board certified professional chaplain. There are no certifying bodies for individual religions. Requirements for APC/BCCI follow national qualifications and competencies common to all chaplains.

In order to become a board certified chaplain through the APC/BCCI, Buddhist chaplain candidates will need an accredited seventy-two-unit educational degree or theological educational equivalency, four units of CPE, and endorsement by a recognized Buddhist community (as described above). In addition, they need to complete one year of chaplaincy employment and essays that demonstrate professional competencies. The first level of competency that the BCCI requires is development and articulation of the candidate chaplain's integration of theory and practice. The second level of competency is the development of professional identity, conduct in relation to others, skills in relation to systems, professional practice, and organizational leadership.

Certificate Programs

Buddhist certificate programs vary from those situated in academic settings to those that offer various forms of Buddhist contemplative caregiver and practitioner training based on the tradition or organization issuing the certificate. Certificate programs may be within a university or college, a nonprofit organization founded by a recognized Dharma teacher with chaplaincy experience, or in partnership with a recognized Dharma center, community, or Sangha. Programs may be part-time, full-time, hybrid, or intensive low-residency models geared toward the adult learner. They aim to enhance skills in pastoral or spiritual counseling, contemplative care, and mental health. Some programs offer specific certificates in Buddhist contemplative care, counseling, ministry, or chaplaincy to professional caregivers in the fields of medicine, psychology, and social work. While a certificate alone is insufficient to meet professional certification standards for educational credits, it may be a wonderful compliment to anyone in a caregiving or helping profession, as well as to train Sangha leaders in pastoral or spiritual care and counseling skills.

Hospice and prison volunteers, Buddhist monastics, priests, and other serious practitioners may also seek to learn basic reflexive listening, contemplative care, and chaplaincy skills to integrate with their Dharma training. Depending on the setting and the leadership, Buddhist chaplaincy certificate programs can be strong in integrating Dharma training, but those outside academic settings often do not provide more academic components. Also, the training by and for Buddhist lineages, often intended for leaders of Sanghas and temples, is not necessarily sufficient for training as a chaplain, which by definition is a religious professional working outside their own religious affiliation or congregation to serve the spiritual needs of all people.

However, some certificate programs are entering into agreements with seminaries or other Buddhist universities to make a bridge for those that would like to build a broader foundation for their service as a chaplain or to complete the academic requirements for APC certification.

Conclusion

There is often a question as to why the MDiv or MA in Buddhist chaplaincy requirements is seventy-two units as opposed to the usual forty-eight units of an MA degree in Buddhist Studies, and why the year-long internship and endorsement processes exist. This relates to the APC requirements, but also to the educational foundation, maturing process, and time necessary to grow into the role of a chaplain. Generally speaking, this development includes not only building a strong theoretical foundation for one's ministry, but also instruction, practice, and training intended to deepen one's faith or spiritual development, as well as the development of the clinical skills necessary to serve wisely and well. This maturing process goes beyond intellectual learning of theories and information. It takes time in an educational program, time practicing as a chaplain in a supervised internship, and time in relationship with a Dharma teacher, mentor, or guide, as well as a Sangha community, to grow into the role competencies of a chaplain.

There are complexities in accreditation, endorsement, and certification. There have already been some cases in which students have been taken advantage of monetarily and misled based on ignorance, miscommunication, the belief that there is an easier way or a shortcut, or trusting a person or institution claiming to offer valid education or endorsement when they were unable to do so. It is very important, as responsible educators and institutions, that degree and training programs as well as endorsers not mislead students or take advantage of their aspirations, time, and money.

At the same time, there is value in having many pathways and not a one-size-fits-all modality. Some Buddhist chaplains may need to get education, clinical hours, endorsement, and certification through more grassroots organizations, and communities or schools without accreditation, or organizations that do not meet the highest standards. A new generation of aspiring Buddhist practitioners are motivated to find right livelihood and serve the world in the roles of Buddhist chaplain, minister, priest, lay leader, or monastic. As educators, institutions, and practitioners seek to develop capacities to serve others, we must continue to strive for high standards that will support the spiritual or ethical development of future Buddhist chaplains and ministers.

This chapter is intended to describe the highest standards of academic education, as well as clinical experience and religious endorsement, needed to prepare Buddhist chaplains to meet care recipients in ways that are mutually beneficial, ethically sound, and from the heart. Those interested in pursuing a career in Buddhist chaplaincy are warmly encouraged to seek meaningful discussions with educational institutions and training programs, and to join others in this emerging field, bringing their compassionate presence to alleviate suffering, so needed in this world.

This chapter was originally published on the Chaplaincy Innovation Lab website and is reprinted with permission.

24

"SUFFERING IS NOT AN EMERGENCY . . . AND, IT MATTERS TO END IT"

Outcomes of Training Tibetan Buddhist Scholar-Practitioners for Professional Spiritual Care

By Leigh Miller, PhD

One day in a large urban hospital in Portland, Oregon, the occupational therapist on an interdisciplinary care team shared her surprising observation of the Spiritual Care Department's two Buddhist chaplains, Carl and Julie. She said, "You're the only ones who are not eager to rush in like the house is on fire. The more chaotic things get, the more grounded you two get." Julie and Carl had not known they were perceived in this way, but agreed it was true. Does this observation suggest there may be something unique about Buddhist chaplaincy or spiritual care, including in response to "crisis"?

I suggest here that Buddhist graduate education, paired with Buddhist spiritual formation, makes the emerging field of Buddhist chaplaincy unique and important. My interest in the ways in which Buddhist graduate education prepares and supports alumni for serving as spiritual care providers is informed by my teaching, students, and colleagues at Maitripa College,[1] and by enriching conversations about Buddhism and spiritual care with chaplains, seminarians, and those in academic, clinical, professional, and research settings.

My hopes for what Buddhist education and spiritual formation for chaplaincy can look like spring from the encouragement of two inspiring teachers. The first is Yangsi Rinpoche's skillful nurturing of Master of Divinity (MDiv) students at Maitripa College. Rather than a curriculum of formulaic reductions of what they should do, he models and cultivates how to be: Graduates embody ways of being that manifest genuinely and creatively in moments of service to others and that arise from their integrated study and practice of Buddhadharma. The second is a question I thank Reverend Dr. Daijaku Kinst for encouragingly keeping before me: How does the heart of Buddhist education root students in a tradition and create a foundation from which to serve diverse others?[2] Yangsi Rinpoche and Daijaku Kinst trust in their graduate student scholar-practitioners' capacity to integrate the teachings and practices of Dharma—the heart of the training—alongside a robust contemporary curriculum's many components. They may thereby embody and express an "appropriate response" toward others in crises or seeking spiritual care from Buddhist ministers or chaplains.[3]

I have informally followed a group of chaplains for two years for glimpses of what this looks like in day-to-day service as a hospital or hospice chaplain.[4] Put another way, how does Buddhist theological education result in and also engender ongoing spiritual formation in spiritual care providers? What do Buddhist chaplains point toward as most significant for their caregiving and crisis care? I share below some of those illustrative moments and the themes that unfolded through listening to their voices. Themes focus on suffering, worldview, relationships, and Dharma practice.[5] First, as the training for spiritual care is critical to subsequent praxis and professional certification, I will very briefly describe the state of Buddhist theological education in the United States today.

Buddhist Graduate Education and Professional Chaplaincy

While chaplaincy-oriented graduate degree programs in the United States focused on Buddhism meet the curricular requirements of the Association of Professional Chaplains, they often also understand "learning" in specific ways. In the Tibetan Buddhist monastic training curricula, "study" and "practice" have been inseparable since the twelfth century.[6] In Tibetan Buddhist schools, the theory of learning exceeds acquisition of knowledge or information and offers a method of increasing subtlety and integration, called the Three Wisdoms. The student first hears or reads the doctrine and grapples with intellectual understanding of the textual content. The student next contemplates or critically reflects on that understanding, examining and testing whether the claims asserted could be verified by one's own experience and reasoning. Finally, the student meditates, with concentrative and analytic methods, upon the subject until it is "realized," a state of doubtless insight that irrevocably changes the meditator's relationship to self, others, and the nature of reality.

This takes place with a mentor, and in community. Study is constituent of being on a spiritually transformative path of liberation for oneself and others. The Tibetan Buddhist lineages intend to produce learning that is not merely intellectual or hypothetical, but experientially grappled with and integrated in order to bring about transformation; this is inseparable from the cultivation of boundless wisdom and compassion toward the liberation of all beings. In graduate education, courses in Buddhist critical constructive reflection draw out the co-construction of philosophy, practice, social institutions, and self that undergirds contemplative pedagogy and learning-centered community at Maitripa College. The result is "spiritual formation."

The heart of Buddhist training may most closely resemble what those in seminaries and spiritual care departments and professional associations refer to as "spiritual formation." Standards for certification in professional chaplaincy and the demands of employers stress the primacy of spiritual formation as a result of graduate theological education and clinical pastoral education. This includes thorough doctrinal study and critical constructive reflection on one's own tradition, self-awareness, and the cultivation of a spiritual maturity comfortable with others' different traditions that is marked by respect, interest, and affirmation.[7] Spiritual formation expresses itself in stable nonjudgmental presence, compassionate deep listening, loving-kindness, equanimity, empathetic joy, generosity, patience, ethical discipline, perseverance, wisdom, and more. Questions that are presently alive in collaborative research among theological school educators, sociologists, clinical pastoral education educators, and chaplain employers include: "What is required most in training chaplains to be able to serve known and emerging needs?" "What is most efficacious?" and "At what locations along the course of training for chaplaincy are these insights and skills developed?"

The need is clear for spiritual formation and graduate education also to embrace understanding of how systemic oppression and racism have for generations traumatized and built resilience within Black, Indigenous, Asian-American, Latinx, immigrant, and LGBTQ+ communities, as well as those impacted by ableism, misogyny, and discrimination. We must be able to serve as allies and advocates for the individuals in our care, within institutions and cultures, and for ourselves, through visibility and skillful insight into intersectionality, privilege, and use of power.

Buddhists have much to contribute to trauma-informed care, antiracist work, and interfaith and secular spirituality with equanimity, compassion, and wisdom. Yet these front lines of spiritual care as it is emerging for the twenty-first century[8] are not specific just to Buddhist spiritual formation. Our world is asking this of all who train for spiritual care, and Buddhists are finding our own language, practice, and doctrinal roots for this work.

Buddhist traditions also have unique contributions to make to the fields of spiritual care, for instance about death and dying, the profound power of compassionate presence, various techniques of deep listening and skillful means, and contemplative practices for cultivating compassion and empathy toward oneself and others. Many others are contributing to this growing interface, which is beyond the scope of this chapter. What I will focus on here is how the heart of Buddhist practice and study in a robust MDiv program (increasingly attentive to the above needs in the United States) manifests in the experience of Buddhist chaplains.

I turn to the voices of fifteen Buddhists to help create some fuller images of what being rooted in Buddhist tradition and practice following graduate school looks like for them as spiritual care providers. Four aspects of Buddhist spiritual and crisis care expressly rooted in particularly Buddhist training that repeatedly arose in our conversations are: (1) the truth of suffering; (2) holding a Buddhist worldview or theological framework; (3) relationships with teachers, Sangha, and enlightened beings; and (4) nourishing and sustaining self-care and Dharma practices. These four aspects of Buddhist spiritual and crisis care are but some of the unique dimensions emerging from the Buddhist voices in my opening conversations and observations with chaplains and clinical pastoral education (CPE) residents. I will explore each in more detail below.

The Truth of Suffering

Let's return to Carl, one of the two Buddhist board certified chaplains mentioned in the opening story, who was complimented for his composure during chaotic times. Carl later reflected that his mode of responding to patients and families comes directly from the Buddha's First Noble Truth, the fact of the omnipresence of suffering for living beings. He explained that, privately, his own theodicy leads him to conclude that "The fact that someone is suffering is not actually an emergency. It's what is happening because of karma and various causes and conditions . . . and it matters to end it." Carl uses Buddhist theological reflection to grasp why we suffer and uses Buddhist practices of compassion and *bodhicitta* to guide what to do about it. He hopes to ensure his presence and interventions with patients focus on their perspective and needs, and how he can support them to alleviate their suffering as much as possible.

If suffering is a Buddhist doctrinal fact, then what is an emergency or crisis? In this, the perspective of the chaplain and patient may be different. The chaplain is there to witness, accompany, and intervene in the patient's crisis. The Buddhist chaplain may be perceived as mindful, centered, or grounded, relative to the panic, fear, chaos, or rushing of others around them. Like all chaplains, they must rely on healthy boundaries, self-care, and self-awareness (including transference and countertransference), to not respond as though they are also in crisis. If and when they are able to bring a compassionate, nonanxious presence into the room where a crisis is unfolding, they make a positive difference. How does the Buddhist chaplain access, cultivate, and hold such presence?

Kate, an MDiv student, reflected after her CPE internship on the relationship between suffering, wisdom, and compassion. She defines wisdom as that "which recognizes everything and everyone as impermanent and even as lacking inherent existence. That informs the Buddhist teaching that we should see all things and experiences as dreams." This is helpful for Buddhist chaplains because:

> It allows us to bear the weight of the suffering we witness. With our hearts wide open to the suffering of another, if we were to see that suffering as more

than it actually is, it would only cause us distress that would prevent us from offering our calm and loving presence. When we see the experience of the suffering person as a dream, it's not that we think they're not suffering or that their suffering doesn't matter. It's that we know their suffering will pass, and we know that their suffering cannot destroy who they truly are in their heart, their goodness. We can have confidence in them, and optimism for them, even as we witness their unbearable pain, even as we let our own hearts break with them, and for them. This allows us to be calm, grounded, and present. Were we to see their suffering as an unacceptable emergency, we would be useless to them. Wisdom into what is really happening allows us to best serve those in our care with compassion.

Mark, an MDiv student eight weeks into his first twelve-week CPE unit, stated,

> When I've seen really deep suffering, someone in really deep spiritual despair, I do feel and I can offer empathy. But there's a deep feeling of recognition that this is where we are [all] at; that you are suffering and this is samsara. I'm attuning to [the patient] but inwardly I remember, in Buddhist iconography, that slight smile on the Buddha's face. There's some feeling of equanimity there. And this has been surprising.

As a Buddhist chaplain in training, he discovered the possibility of being simultaneously deeply attuned to and present with another's despair and also maintaining his own equanimity through recalling the nature of our lives according to the Buddha's teachings.

Prince Siddhartha's Four Sights of the suffering of persons who were sick, elderly, and dead, so the story goes, galvanized his spiritual quest to seek, like the peaceful renunciant whom he also witnessed, the alleviation of suffering and the attainment of awakening. As Buddhist chaplain Anna reflected, "One thing I love about this job is that the teachers of sickness, old age, and death are always present."

The importance of the twin concepts of the pervasiveness of suffering and the potential for liberation from suffering cannot be overstated for Buddhist philosophies. In the Tibetan Buddhist tradition, as is often emphasized by His Holiness the Dalai Lama, all sentient beings desire happiness and to avoid suffering, in exactly the same ways we ourselves do; realizing this, one refrains from harming and increases loving-kindness and compassion toward others as equal to, or even more important than, the self.[9] The unique Buddhist philosophical position that suffering is both pervasive and can be overcome situates the Buddhist chaplain in a specific perspective: able to empathetically and compassionately acknowledge and respond to suffering without being overly avoidant of or consumed by it, knowing it will change, and without unrealistic expectations about our present limitations to effect that change.

In Buddhist spiritual care, the cornerstone motivation to be of benefit to all beings is presumed and expressed in the form of a bodhisattva vow. Yet the keen insight to diagnose the causes of various forms of suffering, discern what will alleviate suffering, and then employ skillful means to offer an appropriate response or path to liberation are all capacities that are developed gradually along the spiritual path until perfected by those having reached Buddhahood. The endpoint of spiritual formation is a lifelong, or a many-lifetimes-long, process to which aspirants on the Buddhist path commit. And yet there is no waiting for perfection before jumping in to do one's best to joyously persevere in study, practice, and service to others. The Buddhist chaplain's path mirrors this, from a motivation to selflessly serve those in crisis to a socially conscious awareness of suffering and the use of various techniques and interventions.

Carl, who's been a full-time oncology chaplain for several years, said:

> We are basically doing acute spiritual care. We get one maybe two visits with patients. We hardly ever see the results of our care and we cannot control outcomes. We can only control the causes we are creating. We can't fix their situation, but I hope that what I offer will bear some fruit down the road.

Of course, what causes can be created—from the professional assessments, interventions, and interpersonal connection Buddhist chaplains offer others, to those seeded in the chaplain's own mind, body, and spiritual practices—and what fruits may ripen look different for each chaplain, but are deeply informed by their Buddhist training. I am struck here by Carl's nonattachment to result or to self, his clear-eyed perspective of worldly and spiritual cause and effect, and the depth of faith in bodhicitta motivation in which it "matters to end" suffering. Carl honestly reflected on suffering, with tears in his eyes, when he said:

> It's ridiculous how much suffering is coming through here day after day; it's like a conveyor belt. It can be really hard because you go through these things with patients and families that are just excruciating. For instance, if a young mother is dying on my floor, that just hooks everyone. The nurses, who see

themselves and their children in her, the doctors, the dietician, the social worker, the CNAs, everyone gets hooked. You can just feel it on the hall, and so that is often what I'm responding to. And then that person dies, and *boom*, up pops another case in the next room, just like it. There's no chance to recover and process and do any of the work people need to do for that because there's the jumping in to the next patient. It can be hard to engage, hold, and move through this suffering.

How does a Buddhist view help chaplains hold such tremendous suffering? Holly invokes the image and story of the thousand-armed, thousand-eyed Chenresig (in Tibetan; in Sanskrit, Avalokiteshvara). She recalls that Chenresig's plunge into

> despair at seeing endless suffering is the moment in which he shatters. But the story doesn't end there; with his mentor's help, he gains eyes to see and arms to extend in helping countless beings. Shedding the illusion of control and having the courage to abandon what no longer works generates richer compassion and empathy.

How we face and work with the despair of ourselves and others matters. Anna, Mark, Holly, Kate, and Carl, as Buddhist chaplains, operate with a recognition of samsara's unceasing suffering and attempt to relate to that fact skillfully, wisely, and compassionately with a potential even for resilience. As Rachel Naomi Remen notes, seeing others as those whom we serve, rather than those who are broken or flawed and in need of our fixing or saving, honors the humanity of our shared suffering, opening space in which intersubjective and relational connections may be accessed for healing and wholeness, and motivates us to contribute to the end of suffering.[10]

Roles of the Spiritual Caregiver Within Buddhist Worldviews

Part of the role of Buddhist theological education and the work of Buddhist educators is to foster learning communities where the "Buddhist emphasis on connecting philosophical reflection to spiritual discipline [flourishes]."[11] As Makransky explains, clarifying and pointing out the connections between Buddhist thought (doctrine) and spiritual exercises (meditation, ritual, *sādhanā*, chanting, and so on) help the student understand the tradition. On this basis, they can then connect Buddhist theological frameworks to their own Dharma practice and to their everyday experiences.

Carl understands his role as a chaplain, working internally and with others in the midst of a "conveyor belt" of suffering, through the paradigm of the four activities of Buddhas. Every action of a Buddha is functionally either pacifying, increasing, magnetizing (the power of attraction), or wrathful (forceful protective means). Most of what chaplains *do,* says Carl, is reducing anxiety, fear, and distress by their presence (pacifying), pointing out and affirming what is going well or strengths present in the patient (increasing), modeling that a spiritual path helps with coping and making meaning of life to inspire others to explore healthy ways of responding to suffering (magnetizing), and holding boundaries if there is a risk present of anyone violating safety or ethical standards through harmful actions of body and speech (wrathful).

Jo, a Zen Buddhist–Sufi hospice chaplain, attributes her Buddhist seminary training with enabling her to see her clients and their families as all located within the infinite and loving expanse of interdependence, through which she channels the already-present sacredness. Vitalia, a Nyingma-trained Tibetan Buddhist hospice chaplain, reflects on her experiences and those of her clients, and all phenomenon, as the nature of impermanence, which she says, "helps with all transitions." For Holly, social justice intersects with Buddhist views: Strong healthy boundaries enable safe practices of keeping her heart open, to "view others' behavior as happening within a larger empathetic framework."

When Buddhist chaplains frame their own being as well as the work they do within a comprehensive worldview formed by Buddhist study and practice, it becomes clear that this framework is larger than cultivating specific qualities valorized by Buddhism (and other faiths), such as compassion and empathy, and more comprehensive than specific techniques, such as presence, deep listening, or skillful means (although these are all also consistently named as essential in their spiritual care). What their thorough training and grounding in their Buddhist tradition offer is this paradigm in which they can locate their spiritual formation and spiritual care to create meaning and purpose, understand multiple scopes of efficacy, and hold a range of mundane to ultimate perspectives regarding the potential and limitations of their internal and interpersonal work, all within samsara and nirvana.

Relationship with Virtuous Beings

A Buddhist framework for spiritual care is enlivened beyond the theoretical and philosophic only through community, with the cultivation of a warm heart and a stable sense of self. Buddhist chaplains generally have established meaningful relationships. Spiritually efficacious relationships, the tradition says, are to be cultivated with Dharma teachers, with Sangha and virtuous friends, and, particularly within a Vajrayāna tradition, with one's lineage, Dharma teachers, and Buddhas and enlightened beings. In many Buddhist contexts, one's Dharma teacher is a supervisor and mentor of scholarly and doctrinal education who is also entrusted by the student or disciple to guide the development of their karma and mind, potentially for the duration of this, or many, lifetimes. Relationship with a teacher and a community may or may not be an integrated dimension of Buddhist graduate theological education, but it is presumed to be established or enhanced by the time a graduate seeks endorsement as a part of the process of board certification as a professional chaplain.

For a unique example, Buddhist theological education at Maitripa College includes strongly integrated philosophy and meditation courses taught by Yangsi Rinpoche, a Geshe Lharampa from Sera Je and Gyume monasteries, who models the generosity, compassion, spaciousness, insight, and wisdom resultant from commitment to his Buddhist training and practice. Students also witness Yangsi Rinpoche's relationship as a student to his own teachers who periodically visit the college; thus they witness the embodying of reliance, trust, altruism, ethics, and warm care between student and teacher that nourishes spiritual formation and enables extending such internal stability and compassionate care for others.

As the journey toward professional chaplaincy continues, Buddhist students undertake CPE, where they are suddenly among others who value being rooted in a spiritual tradition. But in most cases, they find themselves the only Buddhist in the room. They face having to translate their Buddhist immersion learning for a theistic-dominated setting and rely upon their own recollection of the words, presence, inspiration, and instructions of their Buddhist mentors. They discover—in the intensity of their first patient visits, first deaths, first overnight on-call shifts, first patient in crises who reminded them of their own parent or child—that they still possess the strengths, resiliency, and perspective that became so familiar and accessible when they were with their teacher, in community, in the meditation hall, and in their own practice fields. Having experienced reliance and support from Buddhist Sangha while in training, they are able to enter into spiritual friendship with their CPE cohort, in a new facet of their professional and spiritual formation.

In these relationships, particularly with a teacher or in guru yoga meditation, Holly finds the benefit of "growing a spiritually receptive mind," which can be nourished by receiving spiritual care and that recognizes "how much vulnerability and trust others give us when we care for them." Many Buddhist chaplains remark that encounters with those in their care are also a form of "Dharma practice." The care receiver can poignantly stir the spiritual growth of the caregiver when both people feel they are mutual beneficiaries of the gift of spiritual care, making this an important relational aspect of the receptive chaplains' spiritual life.

Ideally, these teachers and Sanghas also offer critical ongoing support to professional chaplains. Jo recalls days when she needs to "nearly crawl on my hands and knees into the Zendo" to just be there without any expectations of her, receiving quiet acceptance and the nurturing presence of teachers and community, even while sitting together in silence. Vitalia invokes the presence of Tara, the female Buddha, "who is always near to me" as comfort, aid, and inspiration. Another chaplain recounted meeting with a close Dharma teacher to complain about the abundance of compassion but dearth of "real wisdom," from a Buddhist perspective, that he finds in the hospital. Yet his teacher revealed a new way to see wisdom in action that is always present. The encounter honored the chaplain's experience while also offering a gentle challenge and perspective shift that fueled many months of increased satisfaction with his job and his practice. Ultimately, what the teacher and enlightened beings model, inspire, and train the student in is not *what* to know, or *how* to respond to specific conditions, but rather *who they can be*. Ideally, the teacher affirms the students' inherent capacity, borne out of integrated study and practice, to offer appropriate response in any situation, *and* gives the student recurring opportunities to receive such spiritual care themselves.

Nourishment and Vitality

Finally, in brief, I want to name as nourishment and vitality that commitment and aspiration Buddhist chaplains express to not burn out, to sustain themselves, and to be able to bring into the room that which they have access to offering *and replenishing.* Burnout, compassion fatigue (a misnomer), and empathetic distress are known challenges in fields of care. At the close of 2020, one Buddhist chaplain told me that her "well had completely run dry, and so has those of all the chaplains in my department." Awareness of the potential for burnout should trigger graduate programs, clinical education programs, and employers to examine their training and cultures regarding the sustainability of spiritual care work for its providers.

There are dimensions of Tibetan Buddhist meditation and ritual practices that are specifically intended to uplift, inspire, and encourage our hearts and minds. While this needs more exploration, I find myself asking this question: What would it look like to emphasize love, rejoicing and sympathetic joy, healing visualizations, and receiving blessing[12] more in our Buddhist seminaries, along with suffering, compassion, confession, and equanimity?

Mark offers an example of how mindfulness helps him remain grounded and open, even when emotions are running high in himself or others, saying, "whenever a strong feeling arises, I can relate to it—to not let it go unnoticed, to know it is an impermanent thought or feeling, and to make a mental note that there's something there to come back to—and also stay connected to caring for the patient for the duration of the visit."

Practices that chaplains access while on the job can be energizing, and at other times, a kind of spiritual treading water or attaching themselves to a buoy on the ocean's turbulent surface. It makes going on somehow possible when one's well feels completely dry, or as another put it, her own emotions feel blunted and connection with patients has become superficial and rote. We must kindly and realistically acknowledge that bringing any internal and spiritual resources to an onslaught of suffering day after day is hard emotional, spiritual, and physical labor. While admirably mindful at work, they also confess to feeling insufficient in their own practice and self-care, too exhausted by a day of work to engage with in-depth, formal Buddhist practice once back home. Somewhat apologetic about how all they can manage are "small" acts of "practice" at work, they long for Buddhist retreats to drink deeply from the well of practice. While hearing this refrain of spiritual longing, I must counter that, of course, it is no small thing to make every moment with those in their care a form of "practice."

Thinking about long-term sustainability, including how it intersects with antiracism work, Holly distilled four views and concordant formation practices.[13] Her definition of sustainable chaplaincy includes longevity, vitality, integrity, and efficacy. Chaplains wishing to cultivate sustainability must practice establishing healthy boundaries, skillfulness in a social justice framework, holding wisely the role of caregiver, and naming the cultures and systems individuals operate within that may cause or hide spiritual wounds. I feel just as importantly, Holly's views and practices for sustainable chaplaincy also include inviting humor and playfulness. In her experience, she finds these through "allowing something unknown to thrive away from the pressures of daily life, intentionally cultivating or training something missing in one's spiritual life or to consolidate and rejoice in one's gains," and enjoying a good meal, poem, or affection with her cat. I imagine the sustainable, nourished chaplain supported in living such that they can access and embody for others joy, beauty, and vitality when they may feel distant from their own.

When Buddhist chaplains shine, they have experienced this vitality. They both receive and provide opportunities to go beyond "maintaining" to a state that genuinely affirms their lives and Dharma practice in profoundly nourishing and joyful ways. Those Buddhist chaplains who spoke to me of their most restorative self-care almost all named Buddhist retreats—days to weeks of dedicated deeper meditative practice, once or more often each year—as essential.[14] Carl finds it healing, after months at a time of swimming in a Catholic hospital in which there is a cross in every room and prayers are closed "in Jesus' name," to go away for immersion in teachings and retreats at a Buddhist center in which he is held in an environment full of Buddhist imagery, and the language of prayer is his own, no translation or code switching required. Without needing to expend energy mediating his environment, his energy is freed up for the practices that directly uplift him. Several chaplains have shared that after meditation retreats, visits with patients are markedly different. Holly said, "I consider retreat an essential sustaining practice in working with experiences of despair as a caregiver." There is easier and lighter access to laughter, tears, authenticity, and transformative accompaniment.

Whether they are in training or years into a professional career, Buddhist chaplains assert the importance of "ordinary self-care" acts that support short-term resourcefulness. It can include play with their dogs or snuggles with the cat, time with poetry or enjoying good food, bike rides, hikes, yoga and dancing, baths, meeting with other Buddhist chaplains or peers, receiving empathy from friends and loved ones, and so on. They distinguish this from the greater resiliency, personal growth, enhanced theological reflection, and blessing that they associate with periodic retreat or significant immersion into their spiritual home practices. We might view such vitalizing combination of self-care and retreat or community Dharma practice for the post-graduate professional chaplain as a reentry into the heart of Buddhist theological education: the spiritual exercises and practices that integrate the tradition into one's relationships, vows, ethical livelihood, theological reflections, and appropriate life-affirming responses.

Conclusion

Mark started a CPE unit unsure about his post-graduate calling. Yet, by the end of the unit, he found himself applying to postgraduate full-time CPE residency programs, the next step on the career path of professional chaplaincy. An even greater surprise for him was, in his own words, "how much I drew on what I learned at Maitripa. Every day." He reflected,

> My time [in Buddhist graduate theological education] has prepared me so well for this work, and I am so grateful for it. I definitely didn't see, during the time I was in coursework, what was happening, but now with some hindsight, I can say, wow, these really are skills that I am cultivating and nourishing, and the fruits are starting to show up a little bit, and it's a really good feeling.

And yet, no graduate theological education program alone could take credit for the spiritual formation and "chaplaincy competencies and outcomes" I celebrate in the Buddhist spiritual caregivers' voices included here. Furthermore, remarks and observations I highlight here have been shared with me in the context of their many years of also addressing—often alone or without the support of their graduate schools, teachers, or clinical supervisors—their own and other's pain from dehumanization, systemic racism, despair, the need for boundaries, gender violence, failures of trauma-sensitive care, exploitation, and exhaustion, sometimes even while in pursuit of the requirements for board certification as a professional chaplain.

Work preliminary to profound spiritual care includes awakening to one's own sociocultural locations, internalized oppression, and complicity with systemic oppression,[15] as well as identifying the spiritual resources to face and transform obstacles to "radical wellness" of self and community.[16] To become part of Buddhist practice and view, insights into the pain of othering must be integrated with complex Buddhist philosophy and practice, which also require years to gain competency, with its pitfalls—especially of spiritual bypassing—and risks. The promise of such work is that the Buddhist chaplain's self is at once protected by professional ethics and boundary-setting, cared for and nourished, and empty of inherent existence in healthy, sustaining ways.[17] This is personal and collective work that, along with nourishing vitality, I believe can and must be increasingly modeled, encouraged, and supported in Buddhist graduate education.

Permit me to close by repeating snippets of Buddhist chaplains' voices that echo in my mind: Suffering is not an emergency, and yet it matters to end it. The teachers of sickness, aging, and death are always present. Equanimity, nonattachment, and compassionate perseverance are possible despite the conveyor belt of suffering. Interdependence, impermanence, and empathy mark socially conditioned life. Virtuous spiritual friends, mentors, teachers, communities, and the presence near to us of enlightened beings: all are actively supporting our well-being, here and now. Our heart-minds—receptive, grateful, humble, wise, tender, joyful—are already enough. . . . May these voices of Buddhist spiritual care providers, and the blossoms of their spiritual formation, perfume the minds, uplift the hearts, and inspire the fearlessness of all who hear them.

NOTES

Introduction

1   Stephen B. Roberts and Willard W. C. Ashley Sr., "Introduction: Disasters and Spiritual Care," in *Disaster Spiritual Care: Practical Clergy Responses to Community, Regional and National Tragedy,* edited by Stephen B. Roberts and Willard W. C. Ashley Sr., 2nd ed. (Nashville, TN: SkyLight Paths, 2017), xv.

2   Stephen B. Roberts and Willard W. C. Ashley Sr., "Introduction: Disasters and Spiritual Care," xv.

3   Stephen B. Roberts and Willard W. C. Ashley Sr., "Introduction: Disasters and Spiritual Care," xvi.

4   Stephen B. Roberts and Willard W. C. Ashley Sr., "Introduction: Disasters and Spiritual Care," xviii. Roberts and Ashley use thirteen points rather than twelve. I included their point number 10 within point number 5 because of their similarity. It was easier to discuss those two points together in the same section.

5   Laura S. Brown, *Cultural Competence in Trauma Therapy: Beyond the Flashback,* 1st ed. (Washington, DC: American Psychological Association, 2008), 4.

6   Thānissaro Bhikkhu, "Mindfulness Defined," Dhammatalks.org, 2, www .dhammatalks.org/Archive/Writings/CrossIndexed/Uncollected/MiscEssays /MindfulnessDefinedOld.pdf.

7   Julie Taylor, "Spiritual First Aid," in *Disaster Spiritual Care: Practical Clergy Responses to Community, Regional and National Tragedy,* edited by Stephen B. Roberts and Willard W. C. Ashley Sr., 2nd ed. (Nashville, TN: SkyLight Paths, 2017), 128.

8   Julie Taylor, "Spiritual First Aid," 133.

9   Jamil Zaki, *The War for Kindness: Building Empathy in a Fractured World* (New York: Broadway Books, 2019), 27.

10 Viktor E. Frankl, *Man's Search for Meaning* (1959; reprinted Boston: Beacon, 2006), 80.

11 Hiroyuki Takamatsu, Akihiro Noda, Akeo Kurumaji, Yoshihiro Murakami, Mitsuyoshi Tatsumi, Rikiya Ichise, and Shintaro Nishimura, "A PET Study Following Treatment with a Pharmacological Stressor, FG7142, in Conscious Rhesus Monkeys," *Brain Research* 980:2 (August 8, 2003), 275–80, doi:10.1016/S0006-8993(03)02987-1.

12 Jamil Zaki, *The War for Kindness,* 102.

13 Stephen B. Roberts, Kevin L. Ellers, and John C. Wilson, "Compassion Fatigue," in *Disaster Spiritual Care: Practical Clergy Responses to Community, Regional and National Tragedy,* edited by Stephen B. Roberts and Willard W. C. Ashley Sr., 2nd ed. (Nashville, TN: SkyLight Paths, 2017), 231–47.

14 Bhikkhu Anālayo, "A Task for Mindfulness: Facing Climate Change," *Mindfulness* 10 (2019), 1926–35.

15 Bhikkhu Anālayo, *Compassion and Emptiness in Early Buddhist Meditation* (Cambridge, UK: Windhorse 2015), 202.

16 See Jamil Zaki, *The War for Kindness,* 35–38.

17 Jamil Zaki, *The War for Kindness,* 178–81.

18 Eve Ekman quoted in Jamil Zaki, *The War for Kindness,* 113.

19 Jamil Zaki, *The War for Kindness,* 112–13.

20 Venerable Master Hsing Yun, *On Becoming a Bodhisattva* (Hacienda Heights, CA: Buddha's Light International Association, 1999), 13.

21 Thupten Jinpa, ed., *Mind Training: The Great Collection* (Somerville, MA: Wisdom, 2014), 560–61.

22 Maria B. Ospina, Kenneth Bond, Mohammad Karkhaneh, Lisa Tjosvold, Ben Vandermeer, Yuanyuan Liang, Liza Bialy, et al., *Meditation Practices for Health: State of the Research* (Rockville, MD: Agency for Healthcare Research and Quality, 2007), www.ncbi.nlm.nih.gov/books/NBK38360. Another significant study in this area was through Johns Hopkins University, which pointed out how most of the forty-seven mindfulness studies in their meta-study had too small sample sizes and design flaws that made the conclusions ambiguous. See Madhav Goyal, Sonal Singh, Erica M. S. Sibinga, Neda F. Gould, Anastasia Rowland-Seymour, Ritu Sharma, Zackary Berger, et al., "Meditation Programs for Psychological Stress and Well-Being: A Systematic Review and Meta-Analysis," *Journal of the American Medical Association, Internal Medicine* 174:3 (2014), 357–68, doi:10.1001/jamainternmed.2013.13018.

23 Funie Hsu, "What Is the Sound of One Invisible Hand Clapping? Neoliberalism, the Invisibility of Asian and Asian American Buddhists, and Secular Mindfulness in Education," in *Handbook of Mindfulness: Culture, Context, and Social Engagement,* edited by Ronald E. Purser, David Forbes, and Adam Burke (New York: Springer, 2016), 369, doi:10.1007/978-3-319-44019-4_24.

24 Thānissaro Bhikkhu, *The Wings to Awakening* (Escondido, CA: Metta Forest Monastery, 1996), 26.

1. The Ecology of the Bodhisattva

1 Allen Ginsberg, Gary Snyder, and Philip Walen, "The Four Bodhisattva Vows," in *Dharma Rain,* edited by Stephanie Kaza and Kenneth Kraft (Boston: Shambhala, 2000), 443.

2 For a discussion of the purification of the buddha-field, see Robert Thurman, *Holy Teaching of Vimalakirti: A Mahayana Scripture* (University Park, PA: Pennsylvania State University, 1976), 111–42.

3 George Sessions, ed. *Deep Ecology for the 21st Century* (Boston: Shambhala, 1995), ix.

4 White as quoted by Warwick Fox, *Towards a Transpersonal Ecology* (Albany, NY: State University of New York, 1995), 5.

5 White as quoted by Warwick Fox, *Towards a Transpersonal Ecology,* 6.

6 White as quoted by Warwick Fox, *Towards a Transpersonal Ecology,* 6.

7 Arne Næss as quoted by George Sessions, *Deep Ecology for the 21st Century,* xi.

8 The first was Næss's description of the philosophical positions of supporters of the Deep Ecology movement as outlined in his 1972 Bucharest paper, the second is Næss's personal philosophical position called "Ecosophy T," and the third is the Deep Ecology Platform developed by Næss and George Sessions in 1984. As Ecosophy T is Næss's personal philosophical position within the Deep Ecology movement, it is not detailed here.

9 Robinson Meyer, "This Land Is the Only Land There Is," *The Atlantic,* August 8, 2019, www.theatlantic.com/science/archive/2019/08/how-think-about-dire-new-ipcc-climate-report/595705.

10 Arne Næss, "The Shallow and the Deep, Long-Range Ecology Movements," in *Deep Ecology for the 21st Century,* edited by George Sessions (Boston: Shambhala, 1995), 151.

11 Arne Næss, "The Deep Ecological Movement," in *Deep Ecology for the 21st Century,* edited by George Sessions (Boston: Shambhala, 1995), 68.

12 "View" (Sanskrit: *dṛṣṭi*) is capitalized here because View is first of the triad, View, Meditation, and Action, when speaking of the Buddhist Path. *Dharma Rain: Sources of Buddhist Environmentalism,* edited by Stephanie Kaza and Kenneth Kraft (Boston: Shambhala, 2000), 4.

13 For an extended discussion on the themes of reverence for life and nature as teacher and refuge, see Stephanie Kaza and Kenneth Kraft, *Dharma Rain,* 14–570.

14 Thich Nhat Hanh as quoted by Sulak Sivaraksa, "True Development," in *Dharma Gaia,* edited by Allan Badiner (Berkeley, CA: Parallax, 1990), 177.

15 For further discussions on these four pairs of dualities see, Karen Lang, ed., *Four Illusions: Candrakīrti's Advice for Travelers on the Bodhisattva Path* (Oxford: Oxford University, 2003).

16 Robert Thurman, *Holy Teaching of Vimalakīrti,* 19.

17 Robert Thurman, *Holy Teaching of Vimalakīrti,* 18–19.

18 Shigen Takagi and Thomas Dreitlein, *Kūkai on the Philosophy of Language* (Tokyo: Keio University, 2010), 117.

19 Dōgen Zenji, "Mountains and Rivers Sutra," in *Dharma Rain: Sources of Buddhist Environmentalism,* edited by Stephanie Kaza and Kenneth Kraft (Boston: Shambhala, 2000), 73.

20 Dōgen Zenji, "Mountains and Rivers Sutra," 21.

21 Robert Thurman, *Holy Teaching of Vimalakīrti,* 19.

22 There are different numbered sets of (close to similar) precepts depending on the various traditions of Buddhism.

23 Robert Aitken, *The Mind of Clover: Essays in Zen Buddhist Ethics* (New York: North Point, 1984), 3.

24 Robert Aitken, *The Mind of Clover,* 3.

25 *Tiep hien,* the two Vietnamese characters for interbeing, carry four aspects, two for each character. They are "being in touch" and "continuation" for tiep, "realization" and "making available in the present" for hien. Fourteen Mindfulness Trainings are based on nonattachment from views, direct experience with meditation, appropriateness, and skillful means. See Thich Nhat Hanh, *Interbeing: Fourteen Guidelines for Engaged Buddhism* (1987, reprinted Berkeley, CA: Parallax, 1998), 3.

26 Padmakara Translation Group, trans., *The Way of the Bodhisattva* (Boston: Shambhala, 2003), 22 (3.22).

27 John Stanley, David Loy, and Gyurme Dorje, eds., *A Buddhist Response to the Climate Emergency* (Boston: Wisdom, 2009), 223–62.

28 The process by which the ego-self is transformed into the eco-self is called greening of self. Macy uses "greening" because the self recognizes its interdependence with nature and nature's nature. Joanna Macy, "The Greening of Self," in *Dharma Gaia: A Harvest of Essays in Buddhism and Ecology,* edited by Allan Hunt Badiner (Berkeley, CA: Parallax, 1990), 63.

29 Macy uses the term *ego-self* to refer to a self that believes in a permanent, independent self. It is in opposition to *eco-self.* This is her term for a "self" that dwells in interdependence with the buddha-ecology.

30 Joanna Macy, "The Greening of Self," 56.

2. Responding to Multiple Crises and the Roles of Community Chaplaincy

1 The Peninsula Solidarity Cohort offers monthly meetings in which leaders and clergy of different faiths come together to be educated by and in dialogue with local nonprofits, social advocates, and other community voices. Other opportunities that emerged from this group have included public speaking, participation in public vigil or ritual, and participating in meetings with local elected leaders, police chiefs, and public health officials.

2 Originally printed in *The Daily Journal,* September 4, 2020. www.smdailyjournal.com /opinion/guest_perspectives/call-for-a-community-ethic-of-compassion/article _11a5e442-ee47-11ea-8890-6f8bf6d3ad91.html.

3 The Depolarization Summit, November 19, 2020, was organized by Millions of Conversations, Vanderbilt University, and the Fetzer Institute. A full recording of the summit is at: www.youtube.com/watch?v=67EymhzqK9A.

4 Sadia Hameed's presentation and model at the Depolarization Summit can be viewed at: www.youtube.com/watch?v=67EymhzqK9A&t=11040s.

5 The Four Great Efforts, as listed in the Pāli Canon, are endeavors of mental cultivation: (1) restraint, to prevent the arising or increasing of unwholesome states; (2) abandonment of arisen unwholesome states; (3) desire for and development of wholesome states such as mindfulness, wisdom, benevolence, compassion, joy, and equanimity;

(4) protection, to protect, maintain, and refine whatever wholesome states have arisen (Anguttara Nikāya 4:14).

6 More detail about social applications of conditionality can be found in this author's MA thesis: Dawn Neal, "Discord and Its Alternatives in the Aṭṭhakavagga of the Pali Canon" master's thesis, Graduate Theological Union, 2017), ch. 5–6.

7 The full formulation of *idappaccayatā* is, "When this exists, that comes to be; with the arising of this, that arises. When this does not exist, that does not come to be; with the cessation of this, that ceases." Bhikkhu Bodhi, trans., *The Connected Discourses of the Buddha: A New Translation of the Saṃyutta Nikāya* (Somerville, MA: Wisdom, 2001), II 21.1.

8 To find organizations and groups involved in addressing armed conflict, bridging social divides, and building community resilience in the United States, see the Bridging Divides Initiative, Princeton University, https://bridgingdivides.princeton.edu /ecosystem-map.

9 Tittha Sutta, Udāna 6.4.

6. Café de Monk: Kaneta Taiō and the Mobile Deep-Listening Café

1 金田諦應 [Kaneta Taiō], 傾聴のコツ [Keichō no Kotsu] (Tokyo: Watekiiki-katabunko, 2019), 31–32. Translation by author.

2 Kaneta Taiō, *Keichō no Kotsu,* 32–33.

3 Kaneta Taiō, "Protecting Life: Suicide Prevention Symposium," Kyoto, 2016.

4 Kaneta Taiō, *Keichō no Kotsu,* 52–53.

5 Kaneta Taiō, *Keichō no Kotsu,* 36–38.

8. Finding Flow in Crisis

1 "Fatal Force: Police Shootings Database," *Washington Post,* www.washingtonpost.com /graphics/investigations/police-shootings-database/.

2 *Oxford Advanced Learner's Dictionary,* s.v. "crisis," www.oxfordlearnersdictionaries .com/us/definition/english/crisis_1.

3 Vajracchedikā Prajñāpāramitā Sutra (Taishō Tripiṭaka 235).

9. Staying Cool During a Code Blue: Caring for a Distressed Fiancée

1 Jean Baker Miller, Judith V. Jordan, Irene P. Stiver, Maureen Walker, Janet L. Surrey, and Natalie S. Eldridge, "Therapists' Authenticity," in *The Complexity of Connection: Writings from the Stone Center's Jean Baker Miller Training Institute,* edited by Judith V. Jordan, Maureen Walker, and Linda M. Hartling (New York: Guilford Press, 2004), 64–89.

2 Maureen Walker, "The Truth About Empathy: It's More Than a Feeling." Maureen Walker PhD, blog, June 2017, https://maureenwalker.com/love/the-truth-about -empathy-its-more-than-a-feeling-article/.

10. A Buddhist Chaplain's Prayer

1 Karl Brunnhölzl, *The Center of the Sunlit Sky: Madhyamaka in the Kagyü Tradition* (Ithaca, NY: Snow Lion, 2004), 74.
2 Thich Nhat Hanh, *The Energy of Prayer: How to Deepen Your Spiritual Practice* (Berkeley, CA: Parallax Press, 2006), 29.

11. Making Friends with the Aneurysm in My Brain

1 Andrew Olendzki, trans., "Skinny Gotami and the Mustard Seed" (ThigA 10.1), Access to Insight (BCBS Edition), November 30, 2013, www.accesstoinsight.org/noncanon /comy/thiga-10-01-ao0.html.
2 Bhikkhu Bodhi, *The Noble Eightfold Path: Way to End Suffering* (Onalaska, WA: BPS Pariyatti, 2000), 1.

12. A Buddhist Counseling Approach for Advanced Cancer

1 Albert R. Roberts, "Bridging the Past and Present to the Future of Crisis Intervention and Crisis Management," in *Crisis Intervention Handbook: Assessment, Treatment, and Research,* 3rd ed., edited by Albert R. Roberts (New York: Oxford, 2005), 778.
2 Ronna F. Jevne, Cheryl L. Nekolaichuk, and F. Helen A. Williamson, "A Model for Counselling Cancer Patients," *Canadian Journal of Counselling and Psychotherapy* 32:3 (1998), https://cjc-rcc.ucalgary.ca/article/view/58607.
3 Allen C. Sherman and Stephanie Simonton, "Family Therapy for Cancer Patients: Clinical Issues and Interventions," *The Family Journal* 7:1 (January 1, 1999), 39–50, doi:10.1177/1066480799071006.
4 Raweewan Pilaikiat, Warunee Fongkaew, Hunsa Payomyong Sethabouppha, Pikul Phornphibul, and Joachim G. Voss, "Development of a Buddhist Spiritual Care Model for People at the End of Life," *Journal of Hospice and Palliative Nursing* 18:4 (August 2016), 324–31, doi:10.1097/NJH.0000000000000255.
5 K. C. Lee and L. K. J. Tang, "Note, Know, Choose: A Psychospiritual Treatment Model Based on Early Buddhist Teachings," *Spirituality in Clinical Practice,* 2021, doi:10.1037/scp0000220. Kin Cheung (George) Lee and Chez Kuang Ong, "The Satipaṭṭhāna Sutta: An Application of Buddhist Mindfulness for Counsellors," *Contemporary Buddhism* 19:2 (July 3, 2018), 327–41, doi:10.1080/14639947.2018.1576292.
6 K. C. Lee and L. K. J. Tang, "Note, Know, Choose."
7 Fernanda F. Zimmermann, Beverley Burrell, and Jennifer Jordan, "Patients' Experiences of a Mindfulness Intervention for Adults with Advanced Cancer: A Qualitative Analysis," *Supportive Care in Cancer* 28:10 (October 1, 2020), 4911–21, doi:10.1007 /s00520-020-05331-1.
8 H. M. Chochinov, D. J. Tataryn, K. G. Wilson, M. Ennis, and S. Lander, "Prognostic Awareness and the Terminally Ill," *Psychosomatics* 41:6 (December 2000), 500–4, doi:10.1176/appi.psy.41.6.500.

14. In the Charnel Ground of a Dying Latinx Man: Practicing with Emilio, El Niño Fidencio, and La Santa Muerte

1 Charnel grounds in India are above-ground sites for the putrefaction of mostly unclaimed bodies that have for millennia been used by members of different religious traditions for spiritual practices. For Vajrayāna Buddhists (especially for Chöd practitioners), these grounds hold important teachings on impermanence and on ways to cut through the fears, fixations, and clingings that routinely disturb our minds. In the modern West, for Vajrayāna practitioners, *charnel ground* is a metaphor for places such as hospitals, prisons, nursing homes, supportive residential housing, and homeless shelters, among many other locations where extreme suffering is often present. As in India, these places are seen as good sites to engage in Chöd and other practices. See Joan Halifax, *Standing at the Edge: Where Fear and Courage Meet* (New York: Flatiron Books, 2018).

2 For information on the history of the noted Mexican miracle worker and healer El Niño Fidencio as well as the practices associated with his cult and church, see Antonio N. Zavaleta, *El Niño Fidencio and the Fidencistas: Folk Religion in the U.S.-Mexican Borderland* (Bloomington, IN: AuthorHouse, 2016).

3 Tonglen is considered a very powerful, secret, and difficult practice in the Tibetan Buddhist tradition. It is recommended that we only engage in this practice after receiving careful instructions by an experienced Tonglen practitioner. In this meditation, we breathe in the suffering of all beings. We breathe in the sufferings of other living beings and use that perception to destroy our self-cherishing mind, which is the source of all our own sufferings. We also breathe out everything we cherish, including our body, possessions, merit, and happiness. We send them toward other living beings for their benefit. Although it is recommended that we do this practice on a regular basis, it is said that it is particularly powerful to do Tonglen when we are facing a serious problem because we can use our pain to develop compassion as well as experience our suffering on behalf of all sentient beings. Some believe that Tonglen practice can heal the practitioner from illnesses. See Lama Zopa Rinpoche, *Bodhicitta: Practice for a Meaningful Life* (Somerville, MA: Wisdom, 2019), 208–16.

4 The Era of the Five Degenerations is a Buddhist teaching about the time when a good eon is finishing and during which many generations of sentient beings live under very difficult conditions. According to the teachings, these adverse conditions have been prevalent since two thousand years ago.

19. Chaplains Need Chaplains Too

1 The full text of "Orphan's Lament" in Khmer, with a recording by Koet Ran and a translation into English by Trent Walker, is available at www.stirringandstilling.org/s07.html.

2 Trent Walker, trans., "Indra's Lute," in Trent Walker, *Until Nirvana's Time: Buddhist Songs from Cambodia* (Boulder, CO: Shambhala, 2022), 29–30.

21. The Heart Consultation Room: Post-Disaster Care and Adapting Chaplaincy in Japan

1 窪寺俊之 [Kubotera Toshiyuki],スピリチュアルケア学概説 [A Survey of Spiritual Care Studies] (Tokyo: Miwashoten, 2008).

22. Aging in China and the Life Care Program of Shanghai Jade Buddha Temple

1 Li Bei, "Provide Warm-Hearted Care for the 'Last Mile of Life': Community Health Service Center 246 in Shanghai," *Labor Watch Newspaper,* November 17, 2020, www.51ldb.com/shsldb/zdxw/content/081c7f87-12c9-40ad-b784-f15e0e71fe29.htm.

23. The Path to Buddhist Chaplaincy in the United States: Academic Education, Religious Endorsement, Professional Board Certification

1 Chaplaincy Innovation Lab, https://chaplaincyinnovation.org.
2 Elaine Yuen, "Faculty Explore Possibilities for Buddhist Chaplaincy in the West," Harvard Divinity School News, March 23, 2017, https://hds.harvard.edu/news/2017/03/23/faculty-explore-possibilities-buddhist-chaplaincy-west; "Education in Buddhist Ministry: Whither—and Why?" video, Harvard Divinity School News, April 23, 2015, https://hds.harvard.edu/news/2015/04/23/video-education-and-buddhist-ministry-whither-and-why; "What Does It Take to Be a Buddhist Minister," video, Harvard Divinity School, May 12, 2015, www.youtube.com/watch?v=4cKqMOnuCbE; How Should We Train Students to Be Chaplains?" video, Harvard Divinity School, May 19, 2015, www.youtube.com/watch?v=Hp2ahUIHp2g.
3 Doug Vardell, "Equivalency Issues for Buddhist Candidates for Board Certification through the Board of Chaplaincy Certification Inc.: A White Paper," Board of Chaplaincy Certification Inc., n.d., https://bcci.professionalchaplains.org/files/equivalency_forms/buddhist_white_paper.doc.
4 Elaine Yuen, "Endorsement for Buddhist Chaplains," *Naropa Magazine,* 2017, http://magazine.naropa.edu/wisdom-traditions-fall-2017/features/upaya-buddhist-ministry.php.

24. "Suffering Is Not an Emergency . . . and, It Matters to End It": Outcomes of Training Tibetan Buddhist Scholar-Practitioners for Professional Spiritual Care

1 Maitripa College (www.maitripa.org) is a Tibetan Buddhist graduate school authorized by the Higher Education Coordinating Commission in the State of Oregon to confer Master of Arts in Buddhist Studies and Master of Divinity degrees.
2 Daijaku Judith Kinst is retiring as the Noboru and Yaeko Hanyu Professor of Buddhist Chaplaincy, Buddhist Chaplaincy Program Director, and Sōtō Zen Buddhist Studies Certificate Program Director of the Institute of Buddhist Studies at the Graduate

Theological Union in Berkeley, California. Kinst wrote about some answers to this question in her wonderful essay, "Cultivating an Appropriate Response: Educational Foundations for Buddhist Chaplains and Pastoral Care Providers," in the pioneering volume *The Arts of Contemplative Care: Pioneering Voices in Buddhist Chaplaincy and Pastoral Work,* beautifully edited by Cheryl Giles and Willa Miller (Boston: Wisdom, 2012).

3 Daijaku Judith Kinst, "Cultivating an Appropriate Response."

4 I thank for their generosity of time and heart, and permission to use their words in this essay, Holly Hisamoto, MDiv, BCC, Hospice Chaplain, Providence Health & Services, 2017–2021; Jo Laurence, MDiv, BCC, Hospice and Palliative Care Chaplain, Providence Health & Services, and Sufi Minister; Carl Jensen, MDiv, BCC, Portland [Oregon] Providence Medical Center; Anna Gammon, Providence Health & Services, Hood River, Oregon; Julie Dreyer, MDiv, BCC, Portland [Oregon] Providence Medical Center; Mark Weidenaar, MDiv, Associate Chaplain, Legacy Salmon Creek Hospital, Vancouver, Washington; Kate Brassington, MDiv.

5 This short chapter's speculations are based on initial interviews, participatory observation, and conversation in 2019–2020 with fifteen Buddhists who were either graduate students in the Buddhist MDiv program at Maitripa College who were in or had completed at least one unit of CPE, or professional chaplains in health-care or end-of-life care settings. I'm grateful to them, and to the editor of this volume, Nathan Michon, for the opportunity to share some preliminary findings.

6 John Makransky, "Buddhist Reflections on Theological Learning and Spiritual Discipline Religious Studies News Published by the American Academy of Religion," *Religious Studies News,* March 2010, http://rsnonline.org/indexa18c.html?option=com _content&view=article&id=77&Itemid=112.

7 In light of Pew Research Center research on the changing landscape of religious affiliation and spiritual belonging in U.S. demographics, it may not be surprising that interest and professions in professional chaplaincy have grown among three populations: those looking for careers related to spiritual meaning outside of traditional congregational settings, those looking for spiritual support in times of crisis, and those institutional employers (hospitals, hospices, prisons, schools, and the military) who recognize unmet needs for professional spiritual care in their clients and hire chaplains. See, for instance, Wendy Cadge and Michael Skaggs, "Chaplaincy? Spiritual Care? Innovation? A Case Statement," Chaplaincy Innovation Lab, 2018, https://chaplaincyinnovation.org/case -statement-summary.

8 For instance, see Cheryl Giles and Pamela Ayo Yetunde, eds., *Black and Buddhist: What Racism Can Teach Us about Race, Resilience, Transformation, and Freedom* (Boston: Shambhala, 2020); David Treleaven, *Trauma-Sensitive Mindfulness: Practices for Safe and Transformative Healing* (New York: W. W. Norton, 2018); Jan Willis, "Race Matters," in *Dharma Matters: Women, Race, and Tantra* (Somerville, MA: Wisdom: 2020).

9 The Tibetan LoJong, or Mind Training, genre of texts and practices, stemming from the Indian Buddhist Shantideva's classic *Guide to the Bodhisattvas' Way of Life* and elaborated in Tibet, should not be understood to promote contemporary fallacies of self-denegrating view, low self-esteem, extreme self-sacrifice, nor be complicit with harmful biases that render some "selves" invisible, and must be read within a nuanced philosophy of the selflessness of all phenomenon. See Thupten Jinpa, *Mind Training: The Great Collection* (Boston: Wisdom, 2006) for his translations of Tibetan texts, and Thupten Jinpa, *A Fearless Heart: How the Courage to Be Compassionate Can Transform Our Lives* (New York: Penguin, 2015) for a contemporary, practical guide to compassion training.

10 Rachel Naomi Remen, "Fixing, Helping, or Serving?" *Shambhala Sun,* September 1999. Reprinted in *Lions Roar,* October 25, 2021, www.lionsroar.com/helping-fixing-or-serving/.

11 John Makransky, "Buddhist Reflections on Theological Learning."

12 Blessing, in a Tibetan Buddhist context, refers to the movement of one's heart-mind in a positive direction, under the condition of an influence of wisdom.

13 Holly Hisamoto, MDiv, BCC, has presented this schema at Maitripa College, Portland, Oregon, in November 2019 and December 2020.

14 Often this requires support from institutions, such as leave and vacation time for retreat, observance of holy days not recognized in mainstream Judeo-Christian and federal calendars, and reforming taxing departmental and institutional cultures that marginalize nontheistic traditions. The responsibility for "self-care" is not the chaplains' alone; institutions, schools, family, and community can all support the sustainability and thriving of chaplains.

15 Karen B. Montagno and Sheryl A. Kujawa-Holbrook, eds. *Injustice and the Care of Souls: Taking Oppression Seriously in Pastoral Care* (Minneapolis: Fortress Press, 2009).

16 Ife Lenard and Ericka Echavarria, "How Can We Be Daringly and Radically Well During Times of Upheaval?" webinar, Center for Contemplative Mind in Society, June 2, 2020, www.contemplativemind.org/archives/5949.

17 This passage intentionally evokes, for Tibetan Buddhist practitioners, both the notion of "preliminary" practices and "self" and "other" teachings. Preliminary practices generally precede permission to engage in some Vajrayāna meditation and ritual practices (Ngöndro), or comprise the opening liturgy of daily meditation or recitation (Jorchö). The genres of teachings that elaborate on the lack of inherent difference between self and other, considered to be profound and advanced teachings, require what Yangsi Rinpoche calls a "healthy sense of self" before it can be responsibly and safely negated according to Prāsaṅgika Mādhyamaka analysis or through the practices of "equalizing and exchanging self and other," first taught by Shantideva in the sixth-century *Bodhisattvacaryāvatāra [Guide to the Bodhisattvas' Way of Life]* and subsequently elaborated in Tibet in the LoJong (Mind Training) genre of texts and practices.

INDEX

National Voluntary Organizations Active
  in Disaster (NVOAD), 5–6
nature
    nature of, 41
    as teacher and refuge, 41
neuropeptides, 17–18
Nhat Hanh, Thich, 13, 41, 43, 96, 97,
  103, 119, 120
El Niño Fidencio, 146, 148–153, 255
Noble Eightfold Path, 7, 9, 26, 57, 187,
  188–189
no-self, 41, 103, 186
Note, Know, Choose model, 131–138

P

Peninsula Solidarity Cohort, 47, 53, 252
Pert, Candace, 17, 22, 27
Platform Sutra, 87
playing, 81, 201–206
polarization, 47, 51–53, 88
post-traumatic growth (PTG), 16
post-traumatic stress disorder (PTSD),
  16, 72, 75, 76
prayer, 115–121
presence
    importance of, 9–10
    trusting, 111–112
promises, avoiding, 11–12

Q

Qin Ling, 216

R

racism, 99–102, 202–203, 236
Rājan Sutta, 50
Ran, Koet, 197
Ratnasambhava, 180
referrals, 15–16
refuge, concept of, 3–4
relationships, cultivating spiritual
  efficacious, 242–243
religious care vs. spiritual care, 211–212
Remen, Rachel Naomi, 240

Right Concentration, 26
Right Livelihood, 223
Right Mindfulness, 9, 26
Right Speech, 11
Rinbutsuken Institute for Engaged
  Buddhism, 70–71, 74–78
Rinsho Buddhism Chaplaincy Training
  Program, 71, 78
rinshōshūkyōshi, 214
ritual, 189–190
Roberts, Albert R., 129
Roberts, Stephen, 4–5, 6, 20
RUST practice, 58–59

S

Sahn, Seung, 95
Saṃdhinirmocana Sutra, 87, 89, 91
Sangha
    formation of, 95
    importance of, 166, 192, 203
La Santa Muerte, 147, 149–153
sati. *See* mindfulness
SDAT (spiritual distress assessment
  tool), 112–113
secondary trauma, 19
self
    greening of, 44–45, 252
    no-self and, 41, 103, 186
    true nature of, 186–187
self-care
    importance of, 114, 245–246
    playfulness as, 205
    in preparation for deep listening, 13
separateness, healing, 91–94
Shanghai Linfen Hospital, 216
signlessness, 103
sinicization, 220
Society for Interfaith Chaplaincy, 214
spiritual assessment, 112–113
spiritual care
    within Buddhist worldviews,
      240–241
    preliminary work for, 247

ABOUT THE CONTRIBUTORS

Noel Alumit is an actor, best-selling author, and Buddhist pastor. He received an MDiv in Buddhist Chaplaincy from the University of the West. His writing has appeared in *Lion's Roar, USA Today, Story Quarterly, McSweeney's,* and many others. He facilitates writing and meditation groups in Los Angeles.

Rev. Dr. Lourdes Argüelles, PhD, LMFT, also known as Lopon Dorje Khandro, was ordained a Ngakpa (lay tantric practitioner) by HE the 8th Garchen Rinpoche and installed as a Lopon (senior Dharma teacher) by HH the 37th Chetsang Rinpoche, head of the Drikung Kagyu lineage of Buddhism in the Tibetan tradition. She is professor emerita of education and cultural studies at Claremont Graduate University in California and a former licensed psychotherapist who worked pro bono with survivors of political torture and with migrants in the US-Mexico borderlands. Lopon Dorje Khandro currently lives in retreat except when teaching at Drikung Kyobpa Choling, a traditional Tibetan Buddhist monastery in Escondido, California, and its Sangha in Latin America.

Stephanie Barnes (Repa Nyima Ozer) has been a practicing Buddhist for thirty-five years. She is ordained in the Repa lineage of the Karma Kagyu school of Tibetan Buddhism, a tradition that trains the mind toward awareness, with attention to what is occurring in the present moment, cultivating an attitude that is nonjudgmental, curious, and kind. Chaplain Stephanie has provided support to interdisciplinary teams in emergency departments and intensive care units in three different hospitals, an all-male prison facility, for fire and medical emergency response teams and, most recently, has worked on a COVID unit throughout the pandemic. Over the last eight years, she has developed and facilitated trauma-informed, body-centered mindfulness practices and wellness support for these various groups. She recently served in northern New Mexico, where she worked in a trauma hospital. Stephanie is now living on the Western Slope of Colorado, where she works as a hospice chaplain.

Alex Baskin is completing a clinical pastoral education residency in order to become an interfaith hospital chaplain. He is a recent graduate of Harvard Divinity School. Alex has lived and worked at the Insight Meditation Society and the Cambridge Insight Meditation Center. For several years, he served as a teaching assistant with a Buddhist studies semester abroad program in Bodh Gaya, India. While in divinity school, Alex supported the research of a multi-institution team that has been comprehensively studying the field of Buddhist chaplaincy. He is a part of a small cohort of new leaders trained by the insight meditation teacher Narayan Liebenson to share Dharma teachings in the community. Additionally, he is a certified leader of the body-wisdom modality InterPlay. Alex also writes poetry, with works appearing in some small-press literary journals. Originally from New Jersey, he lives in Massachusetts.

Dr. g (Claudelle R. Glasgow), PsyD, SEP, NEDA Proficient (doc/we/she) is a multipotentialite serving as healer, author, and educator. As a nonbinary, queer, first-generation Being from Afro-Caribbean-American roots, liberatory views and dismantling constructs naturally flow throughout doc's lineage as well as the work. Dr. g's nearly twenty years in healing are emergent and grounded in a radical existential-somatic approach, which works with the power of the here and now, somatics, creativity, and liberation. doc enjoys the conversations and collaborations that bring difference across diverse streams of thought and ways of being into mutual understanding.

Victor Gabriel is the program coordinator of the Master of Divinity program at University of the West, Rosemead, California. He has taught there since 2010. He has a PhD in Buddhist studies from UWest, a master's degree in Tibetan Buddhism from Naropa University, and a master's equivalent in counseling psychology from Curtin University. His research interests include applied Buddhist "theology"; feminist and queer theory; conceptualizations of the body in Buddhist art; ritual studies and the inculturation of American Buddhism. His practice is to see the classroom as a pure land

and the classroom pedagogy as skillful means while aspiring for wholeness and nonduality between the instructor and the participants.

Anna Gagnon is a board certified chaplain who holds a BA in religious studies and a Master of Divinity in Buddhism. A Buddhist practitioner since 1997, Anna has trained with a wide range of teachers and Sanghas, primarily from the Theravāda tradition. Over the last ten years, Anna has worked as a hospital and hospice chaplain in San Francisco, Denver, and Portland. She now ministers at a small community hospital in Hood River, Oregon.

Jitsujo T. Gauthier is the current chair and associate professor of the Buddhist Chaplaincy department at University of the West. She teaches Buddhist homiletics, spiritual care and counseling, spiritual leadership, and engaged Zen Buddhism for Master of Divinity and Doctorate of Buddhist Ministry programs. Her research focuses on practical application of Buddhism within fields of contemplative education, clinical ministry, and interfaith work. Her dissertation, "An On-the-Job Mindfulness Intervention for Pediatric ICU Nurses," was published in the *Journal of Pediatric Nursing* (2015). She is the author of "Hope in the Midst of Suffering" in the *Journal of Pastoral Theology* (2016), "I Am a Woman: Finding Freedom in Seeing Clearly" in *American Buddhist Woman* (2016), "Formation and Supervision in Buddhist Chaplaincy" in *Reflective Practice: Formation and Supervision in Ministry* (2017), and "Buddhist Chaplaincy in the U.S." in the *Oxford Handbook of Buddhist Practice* (2023). Rev. Jitsujo is a Dharma Holder living in residence at the Zen Center of Los Angeles, ordained within the Zen Peacemakers and White Plum Asanga. She is a member of the Buddhist Ministry Working Group, completed two year-long CPE residencies, and one unit of Certified CPE Educator training. Her practice and pedagogy invite more tenderness and breath into meditation and the classroom.

Chenxing Han is the author of *Be the Refuge: Raising the Voices of Asian American Buddhists* and *one long listening: a memoir of grief, friendship, and spiritual care,* both with North Atlantic Books. She is a regular contributor to *Lion's Roar, Tricycle, Buddhadharma,* and other publications, and a frequent speaker and workshop leader at schools, universities, and Buddhist communities across the nation. Chenxing holds a BA from Stanford University, an MA in Buddhist studies from the Graduate Theological Union, and a certificate in Buddhist chaplaincy from the Institute of Buddhist Studies in Berkeley, California. Her chaplaincy training began in Cambodia and continued in the San Francisco Bay Area, where she completed a yearlong residency on an oncology ward. She is a co-teacher of Listening to the Buddhists in Our Backyard at Phillips Academy Andover and a co-organizer of May We Gather: A National Buddhist Memorial for Asian American Ancestors.

Rev. Hitoshi Jin is the director of the Zenseikyo Foundation and Buddhist Council for Youth and Child Edification and senior researcher at the Rinbutsuken Institute for Engaged Buddhism. Born in Suginami Ward, Tokyo, in 1961, he studied Buddhism at Taisho University and Komazawa University. In 1987 he went to India to study at the Graduate School of Benares Hindu University under the Cultural Exchange Program of the Ministry of Education, Culture, Sports, Science and Technology. This experience provided the foundation for Jin's extensive international relations work in which he has brought critical concepts and practices on Buddhist social engagement to Japan. In his time as director of Zenseiko, he has steered the organization to more critical engagement with human rights issues concerning children while acting as the director of the Childline Support Center. In 2016, he was appointed as the first Spiritual Care Worker to the medical team of Tokyo Jikei University Hospital and Medical School, one of Japan's most prestigious medical schools and hospitals.

Mushim Patricia Ikeda is a core teacher at East Bay Meditation Center in Oakland, California. She entered Buddhism through Korean Zen training in 1982 in Michigan and has practiced widely in a number of related traditions since that time, both as a monastic and as a layperson. As a longtime Buddhist teacher at EBMC, Mushim is called upon to be with those with terminal illnesses, to bless babies, to perform commitment ceremonies, and to perform memorial services. Her original path was art and poetry; Mushim holds an MFA degree from the University of Iowa Graduate Writers Workshop. For more information, see www.mushimikeda.com.

Rev. Dr. Daijaku Kinst is a Sōtō Zen priest and teacher, a core doctoral faculty member of the Institute of Buddhist Studies–Graduate Theological Union in Berkeley, and was named Noboru and Yaeko Hanyu Professor of Buddhist Chaplaincy in 2015. She developed the Buddhist Chaplaincy Program at the Institute of Buddhist Studies and served as its inaugural director. She is author of *Trust Realization and the Self in Sōtō Zen Practice* and many other writings. With Rev. Shinshu Roberts, she is a guiding teacher of Ocean Gate Zen Center in Capitola, California. As a Sōtō Zen priest and teacher, academic, scholar, and author, Daijaku has been committed to studying and supporting authentic and fruitful Buddhist practice for many years. Following her formal priest training, including years at Tassajara, she completed a master's degree in counseling. Her PhD was an in-depth study of Sōtō Zen teachings and how we can create environments in which ordinary complicated humans can realize themselves and serve the world in need. She has taught and led retreats widely, including Gampo Abbey with the Ven. Pema Chödrön, and was appointed International Teacher by the Sōtō School in Tokyo, Japan.

Dr. Kin Cheung (George) Lee is a lecturer at the Centre of Buddhist Studies, the University of Hong Kong, and a founding member of the Master of Buddhist Counselling program as well as the Postgraduate Diploma in Professional Buddhist Counselling program at the center. He received his PhD and MA in clinical psychology from Alliant International University–Los Angeles, MA in marriage and family therapy from the University of Southern California, and MA in Buddhist studies from the University of Hong Kong. Dr. Lee has published in the areas of Buddhist mindfulness, application of Buddhism to psychotherapy, acculturation and family conflicts, and international student psychology. His current research focuses on the appropriation of early Buddhist teachings into a theoretical orientation for mental health treatment. Clinically, he is a California-licensed psychologist, registered clinical psychologist of Hong Kong Associations of Doctor in Clinical Psychology, fellow member of the Asian Academy of Family Therapy, certified therapist in trauma-focused cognitive behavioral therapy, and certified therapist in managing and adapting practice.

Manling Lim is a translator and holistic spiritual caregiver who published a short memoir about her journey in integrative chaplaincy called *Energy of Peace*. She has completed five units of clinical pastoral education (CPE) in addition to a hundred-hour Integrative Chaplain Course incorporating integrative healing modalities into her chaplaincy work. She studied in the Master of Divinity, Buddhist Chaplaincy program at the University of the West.

Rev. Dr. Nathan Jishin Michon is a Shingon Buddhist priest, interfaith minister, chaplain, and scholar. Jishin completed their PhD in religious studies at Graduate Theological Union and MDiv in Buddhist chaplaincy at University of the West. Jishin specializes in crisis and disaster care and completed Fulbright research in Japan, examining the development of Buddhist chaplaincy there since the tsunami of 2011. During Jishin's years in Japan, they cared for tsunami survivors while also traveling the country interviewing leaders of Buddhist chaplaincy programs and observing their different chaplain training courses. Among other works, Jishin is the editor of *A Thousand Hands: A Guidebook to Caring for Your Buddhist Community,* co-author of the *Oxford Research Encyclopedia of Religion* entry on "Buddhist Chaplaincy," and translator of *Providing Presence in the Face of Pain: My Journey into Interfaith Chaplaincy* by Wako Amano. On the side, they are co-director of interfaith ministry education for Unity and Diversity World Council. Jishin has lived in seven countries and previously trained extensively in Zen Buddhism and the Thai Forest Tradition before ordaining within the Shingon tradition.

Leigh Miller, PhD, is director of academic programs and a member of the faculty at Maitripa College in Portland, Oregon. She completed a PhD from Emory University with the dissertation "Contemporary Tibetan Art and Cultural Sustainability," based on ethnographic research conducted with artists in Tibet 2003–2007. She is a member of the Buddhist Ministries Working Group (from 2016), the Buddhist Task Force at the Association of Professional Chaplains (2018–2019), and the Innovations in Chaplaincy Education unit steering committee at the American Academy of Religion (2022–2025). She is a Buddhist mentor for the Chaplaincy Innovation Lab and was a 2020–2021 grantee in their Innovations in Chaplaincy

Education, and completed a unit of clinical pastoral education at Peace-Health Medical Center, Vancouver, Washington. She is working to bring the best of the Tibetan and Western scholastic and contemplative traditions into innovative education, and teaches courses related to contemporary Buddhist thought and socially engaged Buddhism, research in Buddhist studies, and Buddhist spiritual care. She is focused currently on fostering within students—and articulating in the fields of spiritual care—the role of contemplative spiritual formation based on a worldview of limitless human positive potential for sustainably, ethically, and justly meeting the world's sufferings with compassion, love, resilience, and joy. https://maitripa.org/leigh-miller.

Dawn Neal, MA, is an Insight Meditation teacher, practitioner, and Theravāda Buddhist scholar. She works as an interfaith spiritual care professional (chaplain). Dawn also offers coaching to support health-care workers, caregivers, and other professionals in connecting and embodying a sense of purpose, vision, compassion, and joy. For more about her coaching practice, visit https://dawnneal.net. Her teaching schedule is available on her Dharma website, https://liberatingdharma.org.

Chun Fai (Jeffrey) Ng is a graduate of the Master of Buddhist Counseling program at the Centre of Buddhist Studies, University of Hong Kong, and a certified mindfulness teacher with the Search Inside Yourself Leadership Institute. He also holds a Bachelor of Business Administration (Professional Accountancy) from the Chinese University of Hong Kong and is a CPA, CFA charter holder, and certified FRM. His academic areas of interest include Buddhist counseling, mindfulness and Buddhist meditation, contemporary Buddhist practice, transpersonal psychology, and comparative spirituality.

Rev. Dr. Hojin (Hye Sung) Park is a Won Buddhist minister, Dharma chaplain, and faculty at Won Institute of Graduate Studies. Hojin is her Buddhist name. She obtained her doctorate degree in pastoral counseling at Loyola University in Maryland and her master's in applied meditation studies at the Won Institute of Graduate Studies. She earned her undergraduate degree and master's degree from Wonkwang University in Iksan, South Korea, with a major in Won Buddhist studies. Rev. Park has taught

Buddhist pastoral counseling and Won Buddhist scriptures to students at Won Institute. She has been working as a Buddhist student spiritual adviser at Swarthmore College and the University of Pennsylvania.

Rev. Shushin R. A. Peterson is a board certified chaplain and priest in the Sōtō-shū tradition of Zen Buddhism. After spending nearly a decade in China and Taiwan, he served as an active duty Hospital Corpsman and Buddhist Lay Leader in the US Navy before attending seminary and receiving ordination at Sozenji Buddhist Temple, Montebello, California. He now serves as the palliative and hospice spiritual care coordinator at the VA Loma Linda Medical Center. He has provided religious services at Marine Corps Recruit Depot, San Diego, as a community clergy volunteer for several years and continues serving the congregation of Sozenji Buddhist Temple.

Dian "Dee" Sutawijaya is a certified nurse assistant at an assisted senior living facility in Grand Rapids, Michigan, and on a path to becoming a licensed practical nurse in the future. She is a seven-time employee of the month at her facility and emphasizes kindness, compassion, and empathy in both her nursing and teaching. Dee enjoys caring for and connecting with dying residents with patience and compassion to give them their best possible comfort and care during their final days. She came to Michigan from Indonesia, where she was a Buddhist studies teacher for K–12 students for eleven years. Taking care of her gravely ill grandmother then influenced her career changing to nursing, though she loves how both fields have the opportunity to impact the lives of individuals they encounter. Dee likes to enjoy a cup of coffee in local coffee shops, swimming at the pool, sunbathing at the beach in the summer, and hanging out with her friends on her days off.

Rev. Dr. Taniyama Yōzō is a professor at Tohoku University in Sendai, Japan, and helps lead the university's Interfaith Chaplaincy training program. Among numerous other works, he is the author of *Iryōsha to Shūkyōsha No Tame No Supirichuaru Kea [Spiritual Care for Medical and Religious Professionals]*. He serves on the board of the Japan Society for Spiritual Care, the Japanese Society for Hospice and Home Care, and the Japanese Association of Clinical Research on Death and Dying. He is the Secretary-General for the Society of Interfaith Chaplaincy in Japan, and the president of the

Professional Association for Spiritual Care and Health. Taniyama previously worked as a Buddhist hospice chaplain in Nagaoka-nishi Hospital's hospice ward, which was Japan's first Buddhist hospice ward. He also previously worked as an associate professor at Shitennoji University and as a grief care chief researcher with Sophia University. He was born to a temple family in Ishikawa Prefecture and ordained as a priest in the Jōdo Shinshu Higashi-honganji (True Pure Land) Buddhist tradition.

Vimalasara (Valerie Mason-John), Hon.doc, MA, was ordained into the Triratna Buddhist Community in India 2005. They are a senior Dharmacarani, training and ordaining those who identify as women. They are author and editor of ten books including the award-winning *Eight Step Recovery: Using the Buddha's Teachings to Overcome Addiction; Detox Your Heart: Meditations for Healing Emotional Trauma;* and *Afrikan Wisdom: New Voices Talk Black Liberation, Buddhism, and Beyond.* They are the co-founder of the accredited course Mindfulness Based Addiction Recovery (MBAR) and work as an international public speaker and trainer in the field of mindfulness approaches for addiction and trauma. They are one of the founding facilitators of Dr. Gabor Maté's Compassionate Inquiry (CI), a yearlong training, and have a private practice incorporating CI and Internal Family Systems IFS.

Wang Fengshuo, MTS from Harvard Divinity School, is now a researcher of the Center for the Studies of Humanistic Buddhism in Jade Buddha Temple and Dean of Shanghai Juequn Academy of Classical Education. Her research interests include Buddhism, spiritual care, and transpersonal psychology.

Rev. Acala Xiaoxi Wang, MDIV, is an ACPE Certified Educator Candidate and full-time staff chaplain at New York Zen Center for Contemplative Care since 2021. She is also a Chinese immigrant, lay Buddhist, Chinese chaplaincy educator, and translator. Acala received her lay Buddhist minister initiation as a Dhammacari from Dharma Vijaya Buddhist Vihara, where her Dharma name, "Acala," was given. Her minister ordination is also endorsed by the Mid-America Buddhist Association. Acala has a Master of Divinity in Buddhist chaplaincy from University of the West. She completed her clinical pastoral education residency with Stanford Health

Care and served as an interfaith chaplain there prior to joining the New York Zen Center. Acala's educational leadership experiences include serving as a Chaplaincy Educator for Beijing Ciyuan Center of Chinese Association for Life Care, a Buddhist chaplain for Calipatria State Prison, and a Dharma teacher for BOCA Dharma Seal Temple. Acala's contemplative experiences include being a meditation practitioner since middle school age and a resident at two Buddhist monasteries. She enjoyed walking in giant sequoia forests and along the Pacific coast for fourteen years while living in California. As Acala relocated to Manhattan, she has been appreciating all the beauties of four seasons that the city has to offer.

Rev. Dr. Elaine Yuen is an educator and chaplain. She received her chaplaincy training at Thomas Jefferson University Hospital in Philadelphia and is ordained as Upadhyaya (Buddhist minister) within the Shambhala Buddhist community. As a Professor at Naropa University in Boulder, Colorado, she taught courses on pastoral caregiving, contemplative arts, and Buddhist studies between 2012 and 2020. Presently living in Philadelphia, she continues to be involved in chaplaincy research and training. She loves to contemplate how we shape our social interactions with caring, creativity, and mindful presence. Her website on contemplative chaplaincy can be found at http://elaineyuen.com.

About North Atlantic Books

North Atlantic Books (NAB) is a 501(c)(3) nonprofit publisher committed to a bold exploration of the relationships between mind, body, spirit, culture, and nature. Founded in 1974, NAB aims to nurture a holistic view of the arts, sciences, humanities, and healing. To make a donation or to learn more about our books, authors, events, and newsletter, please visit www.northatlanticbooks.com.